Diet-Free for Life

Diet-Free
for Life

A Revolutionary **Food, Fitness,**
and **Mindset Makeover** to
Maximize Fat Loss

Robert Ferguson, MS, CN

A PERIGEE BOOK

A PERIGEE BOOK
Published by the Penguin Group
Penguin Group (USA) Inc.
375 Hudson Street, New York, New York 10014, USA
Penguin Group (Canada), 90 Eglinton Avenue East, Suite 700, Toronto, Ontario M4P 2Y3, Canada
(a division of Pearson Penguin Canada Inc.)
Penguin Books Ltd., 80 Strand, London WC2R 0RL, England
Penguin Group Ireland, 25 St. Stephen's Green, Dublin 2, Ireland (a division of Penguin Books Ltd.)
Penguin Group (Australia), 250 Camberwell Road, Camberwell, Victoria 3124, Australia
(a division of Pearson Australia Group Pty. Ltd.)
Penguin Books India Pvt. Ltd., 11 Community Centre, Panchsheel Park, New Delhi—110 017, India
Penguin Group (NZ), 67 Apollo Drive, Rosedale, North Shore 0632, New Zealand
(a division of Pearson New Zealand Ltd.)
Penguin Books (South Africa) (Pty.) Ltd., 24 Sturdee Avenue, Rosebank, Johannesburg 2196, South Africa
Penguin Books Ltd., Registered Offices: 80 Strand, London WC2R 0RL, England

While the author has made every effort to provide accurate telephone numbers and Internet addresses at the time of publication, neither the publisher nor the author assumes any responsibility for errors or for changes that occur after publication. Further, the publisher does not have any control over and does not assume any responsibility for author or third-party websites or their content.

First edition: January 2011

Library of Congress Cataloging-in-Publication Data

Ferguson, Robert.
  Diet-free for life : a revolutionary food, fitness, and mindset makeover to maximize fat loss / Robert Ferguson.—1st ed.
    p.   cm.
  Includes index.
  ISBN 978-0-399-53636-6
  1. Weight loss. 2. Reducing diets. I. Title.
  RM222.2.F4268 2011
  613.2'5—dc22   2010035146

PRINTED IN THE UNITED STATES OF AMERICA

10   9   8   7   6   5   4   3   2   1

Neither the publisher nor the author is engaged in rendering professional advice or services to the individual reader. The ideas, procedures, and suggestions contained in this book are not intended as a substitute for consulting with your physician. All matters regarding your health require medical supervision. Neither the author nor the publisher shall be liable or responsible for any loss or damage allegedly arising from any information or suggestion in this book.

The recipes contained in this book are to be followed exactly as written. The publisher is not responsible for your specific health or allergy needs that may require medical supervision. The publisher is not responsible for any adverse reactions to the recipes contained in this book.

Most Perigee books are available at special quantity discounts for bulk purchases for sales promotions, premiums, fundraising, or educational use. Special books, or book excerpts, can also be created to fit specific needs. For details, write: Special Markets, Penguin Group (USA) Inc., 375 Hudson Street, New York, New York 10014.

To my wife, Krista, and my daughters, Felicity and Faith

Writing a book can be overwhelming for one's family. I'd like to thank mine for their patience and understanding throughout this process. Putting off family time and having to miss some play times has been the most difficult part of this process, but now it's done, and the play times are even more appreciated.

Acknowledgments

I'd like to thank my publisher, John Duff, and the Penguin Group for this opportunity to help others get off the diet merry-go-round. In addition, I want to acknowledge my book agent, Alex Fields, and my manager and friend, Steve Allen, for connecting the dots and helping make this book a reality.

Also, a big thank-you to Provida Life Sciences (Alchemy Worldwide), with which I codeveloped the Food Lovers Fat Loss System—making it possible for people to experience my Metabolism Makeover and sustainable fat loss principles. My relationship with Provida Life Sciences made it possible for me to quickly enter the homes of millions of people who have now embraced my philosophy and the science of eating real food while losing real pounds. As well, I'd like to thank Jusuru International for their support of this book and for giving me an opportunity to work with them on this revolutionary fat loss and metabolism-friendly program.

A big shout-out to my assistant and right hand, Briana Mackey, who spent hours helping me turn out delicious and nutritious recipes for this book. Also major thanks to Randa Dinkler for proofreading and helping to bring clarity to my message, and to my executive assistant and our director of nutrition at the Diet-Free Life Clinic, Brandy Beesley, for her assistance in helping me help others.

My appreciation to Judy Kern, who helped me write this book and make it a good read as well as an invaluable and easy-to-follow guide to health and fitness.

And finally, thanks to my mother, Brenda A. Watson, who has offered me constant and much appreciated feedback throughout this process.

Contents

Foreword

I first heard about Robert Ferguson in early 2005, when he was featured in a health and wellness publication in our local community. As a physician, I am always in search of resources that can empower my patients to win the long-term battle with excess weight, and I was intrigued with both his philosophy and his approach to weight loss. He was obviously knowledgeable about nutrition and fitness, but even more important, he advocated a strategy that would allow people to live leaner and healthier for the long haul.

After meeting Robert and seeing his work firsthand for several years, I can truly say that he is a gifted coach and motivator who is committed to helping people around the globe live *Diet-Free for Life*. If you follow the advice Robert has provided in this book, I guarantee that your outlook and approach to weight loss and weight maintenance will be changed forever. You will achieve lasting weight and fat loss success! You will no longer be searching for the next greatest weight loss pill or diet. Instead, you will be transformed and empowered to control your own destiny in regard to your weight.

Diet-Free for Life is not a gimmick. This is the real deal, leading to lasting weight loss success.

—David P. Pryor, MD, MPH

The Promise of Living Diet-Free

If you've been gaining and losing weight over and over for most of your life, I can appreciate what that's like. I'm no stranger to the joy of losing weight and the pain of yo-yo dieting.

Over the years, I've watched as my mother gained and lost an estimated 1,600 pounds. I was there when she celebrated losing 100 pounds on a low-calorie liquid diet and when she gained back all those unwanted pounds plus a few more. I cheered when she lost more than 100 pounds on a low-carbohydrate, high-protein diet, and I felt her pain and embarrassment when those pounds came back. Seeing so much effort come to nothing again and again was bitterly disappointing for her and heartbreaking for me to watch.

I realize that my mother is not the only one wrestling with these issues. Too many men and women are fighting weight gain and losing the battle no matter what diet they are following. At any given time, statistics show that two-thirds of Americans are on a diet, and less than 5 percent of the people who actually lose weight are able to keep it off once they stop dieting. And, yes, I have fought the fat loss battle myself.

When I was in the Marine Corps, living away from home for the first time, McDonald's became my home away from home. At the risk of sounding outrageous, I want to be candid with you and share exactly what I ate every day. For both lunch and dinner I would order and consume one Big Mac, one cheeseburger, one large and one small order of fries, a hot apple pie, a caramel sundae with nuts, a large strawberry shake, and a large diet soda. Sometimes I'd also add a small box of cookies to my order. Needless to say, it didn't take long for my overindulgence to start showing up on my body. Lucky for me, my Marine Corps camouflage made it easy to hide my heft.

One day, while I was relaxing in front of the television, digesting my latest McDonald's meal, a friend took my picture. When I saw the print a few weeks later, I was shocked. How could I have gotten so fat in so little time?

I was scheduled to go home on leave a couple of months after that, but I immediately phoned my mother and told her that I'd had to change my plans. There was no way I was going to go home looking the way I did. Without realizing it, I had stumbled into the same trap my mother and so many others were trying to break out of—fighting unwanted fat.

I was determined to win this fight, so I began doing what I felt would work. I quit McDonald's cold turkey and started eating foods I thought were healthier, even if I didn't particularly like them. But my immediate instinct was that I needed to start moving. "Run, Robert, run" became my mantra. I ran often: first thing in the morning, at lunchtime, and before going to bed. My strategy worked, and in a relatively short time I was back to a lean 170 pounds.

That was all well and good, but I still had a problem: Was I going to have to run three times a day and eat food I didn't really like for the rest of my life just to avoid being fat? If so, I didn't think this was a lifestyle I was going to enjoy or could even sustain.

With time I've come to realize that it wasn't actually *what* I was eating at McDonald's that was to blame for my weight gain; it was actually *how much* food I was consuming at every meal. My way of eating was definitely excessive, but dieting was not something I wanted to do. To me, dieting meant restriction and denying myself the foods I really liked. And that's what it means to most people. Since those early days, however, I've learned that it is not only possible but actually *easy* to reduce your waistline without having to adhere to a strict "diet." You can lose weight eating the foods you normally eat and love—at home, in fine-dining restaurants, and even at McDonald's.

If you are one of the lucky ones who has never been forced to diet (or has done so only infrequently), I am happy that you've come to this book before you fall prey to a lifetime of going from one weight loss diet to the next. And if you have already been on the diet roller coaster, I hope that what I have to offer will bring that nerve-racking ride to an end.

As I explain the psychological and physiological relationships among food, mood, and fat loss, I will also share the inspiring stories of people, including my mother, who have been able to lose more than 100 pounds following the nutrition and exercise science outlined in this book without ever feeling deprived, restricted, angry, or guilty during the process.

I want you to win at fat loss, and this book is going to provide you with what I believe are the three truest determinants for losing weight and keeping it off for a lifetime: (1) food, (2) fitness, and (3) mindset.

1

You Can Live Diet-Free

Insanity: doing the same thing over and over again and
expecting different results.
—ALBERT EINSTEIN

You don't have to be an Einstein to see that managing one's weight
is an ongoing challenge around the world. And it will continue to be a problem
until we change the attitude that created it and embrace the concept of a diet-
free life.

WHAT IT MEANS TO LIVE DIET-FREE

To live a diet-free life means not feeling restricted or deprived in regard to
what you can or cannot eat. It means not thinking "I have to but I can't" or "I
can't but I have to." It's about how you *think* just as much as it is about how you
eat or exercise. It involves combining practical nutrition information and an
active lifestyle with a mindset that keeps you motivated.

A Diet Mentality Says: I must deprive myself of food or must exercise to
excess in order to lose weight.

A Diet-Free Mentality Says: I can lose weight eating whatever I want so long
as I do it in a way that will provide my body with adequate nutrition and keep
my blood sugar from fluctuating too high or too low.

EMBRACE THE POSSIBILITY THAT IT'S POSSIBLE

You can eat a burger and lose weight. You can have bread and release fat. You can eat fruit and shed inches. You can even drink a regular soda and drop pounds. If you think this is too good to be true, you'll probably prove yourself right. However, if you think it might be true and you're looking forward to the opportunity to try, you're also right. The way you are going to change your mindset is by learning something new about nutrition and exercise, putting that knowledge into action, and experiencing the results. As well, with your newly acquired knowledge, it is also important to acquire the skills that make it easier for you to upgrade your mindset and apply what you have learned.

When Esther B. came to me carrying an extra 60 pounds, she couldn't accept the idea that she could eat burgers and bread, drink regular soda, and still lose weight. It contradicted everything she believed about weight loss. Her mental attitude was that if you want to lose weight, you must stop eating the foods and drinking the beverages that caused you to gain the weight in the first place. She simply couldn't wrap her mind around the possibility that she could lose weight differently than the way she'd been trying in the past. But it took only seven days for her to see results, which enabled her to embrace the new mindset that ultimately led to her losing those 60 extra pounds while still maintaining her close relationship with burgers, bread, and soda.

THE BIG QUESTION: WHY DO YOU WANT TO LOSE THE WEIGHT?

To really adopt any kind of change, you first need to have a good reason for doing it. Your motivation is going to be the driving force that propels you to take action, lose weight, and become diet-free. For my client Sherry G., that motivation was the desire to feel good about her body and her appearance. She had outfits she wanted to wear and loved shopping for new clothes. You might think that wanting to improve your appearance and wanting to buy new outfits are too shallow to be good motivators, but the truth is that there is no right or wrong motivation, so long as it ignites and fuels *your* fire.

SET A REALISTIC GOAL

You might consider yourself to be the most motivated person in the world, but if your desire is to achieve an unrealistic goal, it's not going to happen. I've found that many of my clients have been trying to reach an unrealistic goal weight because they've accepted conventional standards for what they *should* weigh, which are based on incomplete information. Sherry, for example, had been told that to attain her healthy goal weight, as determined by the body mass index (BMI), she needed to lose 60 pounds. But, as I explained to her, there is a more accurate way to calculate healthy weight—one that takes into consideration not only scale weight but also body composition—and based on my calculation, she really only needed to lose 35 pounds. (Read more about healthy weight in Chapter 4.)

For Sherry, the difference between 60 pounds and 35 pounds was monumental. For the first time in her life, reaching her goal weight didn't seem impossible. Keeping her eye on that goal removed a huge mental obstacle and gave her the will to make the goal a reality.

Having a clear, specific, and *realistic* goal can make the difference between success and failure. When you know *where* you're going and believe that you will get there, you become better able to dispel doubt, worry, and the fear of failure.

LEARN THE TRUTH ABOUT NUTRITION AND WEIGHT LOSS

By educating yourself about how your body processes food, what makes you hungry, what makes you feel full, and why it's so important to keep your blood sugar from rising too high or falling too low, you'll have the knowledge to power your eating plan and tailor it to your own needs. Generally speaking, when we understand *why* something works, and it makes sense, we'll be much more likely to do what it takes.

The key to losing weight, staying lean, and being diet-free is learning how to combine an adequate amount of protein with the proper quantities of "fast carbs" and "slow carbs" so that your blood sugar never rises too high, and to snack between meals so that it never drops too low.

GET MOVING TO KEEP LOSING

You can boost your metabolism even more by simply adding daily exercise. This doesn't mean hours in the gym or miles on the road, but it does mean a dedication to establishing an effective exercise plan that works—and works for you. And before you know it—within just 21 days—you will be fully committed to living the diet-free mindset.

THE 21-DAY MINDSET MAKEOVER

The secret to living diet-free is sustaining a lifestyle that works. It is not a one-shot deal; everything you do has to lead you to this fundamental change in the way you *think* about the food you eat, the exercise you do, and the way you live your whole life. The core of this book is the 21-Day Mindset Makeover—21 days of motivation, education, and inspiration that will set you up for a lifetime of good health. The innovative approach offered in this book is called Fresh Start, which is neither a regimented program of deprivation nor a test of your willpower. Rather, it shows you how to make a few simple changes in the way you eat to get results in as few as 7 days—results that will become an essential motivator to the next 7 days and the 7 days after that. And if, as many psychologists attest, a habit can be ingrained in anyone in just 3 weeks, you will be on your way to living diet-free for life.

In the following chapters, I'll walk you through all of it—determining your motivation and your goal, and taking the steps to make over your thinking and your lifestyle so that you, like my thousands of clients, will be living diet-free forever.

▶ The Diet-Free Life in a Nutshell

THE PATH TO living diet-free is simple but not always easy. Knowing what it takes to achieve the goals you seek is the first step.

- Commit to changing the way you think about losing weight and keeping it off.

- Embrace the possibility that a new approach to weight loss will work.
- Find your motivation.
- Set realistic goals.
- Acquire new knowledge about nutrition.
- Learn how to eat the foods you love to maximize fat loss.
- Start to move more to maximize metabolism.
- Keep working on your Mindset Makeover.

2

Set Your Intention

If I can eat all that (and lose weight), sign me up.
— RODNEY PERRY

What motivated you to pick up this book? What are you hoping to get from it? I have to assume that you're hoping to get what I promise: a makeover opportunity for your mindset, an education in nutrition, and a Fresh Start that will allow you to drop up to 7 pounds and shed up to 7 inches in the first 7 days without having to give up all the foods you love.

We all value the idea of losing weight and getting healthier without having to go hungry or eat foods we don't like. But as I've been traveling around the country speaking to many different people, I've come to realize that most people are having a hard time believing that they could possibly lose weight and still enjoy a diet-free life.

If you are one of those nonbelievers, all I'm asking you to do right now is embrace the concept that the diet-free lifestyle you are going to learn about in this book *could* work, and then take the next 7 days to prove to yourself that it does. Set the intention that for those 7 days you will continue to read this book and implement the tools and strategies it offers. And make a further agreement with yourself that when—not if—at the end of that time, you see it *is* working, you will continue your diet-free journey.

You may be motivated to lose weight, but if you don't believe that the process I offer will help, it is going to be difficult for you to put it into action.

That's why I'm asking you to take it on faith and experience it so that you can prove to yourself that it does work.

IF, NOT WHEN

I also ask that you replace the word *if* with *when* in your thoughts and your words. Instead of thinking and saying, "*If* it works . . ." I want you to say, "*When* it works . . ." because there is power in affirming what you want to come to fruition. I'm not asking you to walk around waving your arms and telling everyone you meet how excited you are to shed inches and get rid of unwanted body fat. I am simply asking you to be positive, because being positive sets you up for success and keeps you moving toward your ultimate goal.

TAKING STOCK OF YOUR MOTIVATION

Since you must already be motivated to some degree, or else you wouldn't be reading a weight loss book, I would like you to really examine that motive. It needs to be both strong enough to carry you through to your initial goal and flexible enough to take you to the next level.

Jocelyn C., for example, was motivated to lose weight because she was getting married in 4 months and wanted to look her best for her wedding. She had a *goal* and the *motivation* for achieving it, and I knew that combination would ensure her success. In fact, Jocelyn did lose almost 50 pounds before her wedding day, but then she gained it back. Why? Because once she lost the weight and got married, she lost her initial motivation and never established a *new* goal that would reinforce the success she had found in transforming her body.

Fortunately, Jocelyn contacted me again about 2 years after she had gained all the weight back. I discussed with her the distinction between being motivated and having a goal and helped her to understand that motivation is the "why," the reason for wanting to achieve the goal. A goal is nothing more than a realistic and clearly defined destination. Once you reach your destination (goal), it is important to establish a *new* goal, which is again fueled by the reason (motivation) you want to achieve it.

Jocelyn's new goal was to lose 60 pounds at a rate of 10 pounds every 4 weeks, and her motivation was to feel better about herself—physically and emotionally.

She was fed up with feeling like a failure, feeling tired all the time, and having to settle for wearing her "fat" clothes. So she set her mind on positive emotions: to feel good about herself and her body. Within 5 months it became evident that her motivation was real because she lost the 50 pounds she'd regained plus another 10, and established another new goal to lower her percentage of body fat every 8 weeks until she reached an athletic 18 percent body fat.

To keep moving forward, you need to constantly find new reasons for doing what you're doing or else you'll simply stop doing it. Over time, as you continue to find those reasons, you will experience a mental paradigm shift, and your motivation will go from being *extrinsic* (I do it for x and y reasons) to being *intrinsic* (simply the way you live your life).

EMBRACE AN ATTITUDE OF GRATITUDE

For me, embracing an attitude of gratitude means focusing on what you want to bring into your life instead of what you want to avoid, and then doing whatever it takes to achieve the goal you have in mind. Gratitude simply means being thankful throughout the process.

Most people I have talked to focus on what they *don't* want to come into their lives—"I don't want to get diabetes," "I don't want to shop in the plus-size department," or "I don't want to get a heart attack." This is what I call putting out negative energy. To exude positive energy, focus on the positive reasons behind your goal—"I am reaching my ideal body weight," "I am becoming healthier," or "I am becoming stronger and increasing my energy." That's positive motivation.

Winston Churchill said, "A pessimist sees the difficulty in every opportunity; an optimist sees the opportunity in every difficulty." Patricia C., who had been a client on and off for years, was without question a pessimist who consistently focused on what she didn't want instead of what she did want, until one day she experienced a true Mindset Makeover. Instead of coming to our coaching session assuming, as she would have in the past, that she hadn't lost any weight, she arrived with a positive attitude and focused on how she could get the most out of her time with me.

When I asked her what had changed, she said that she'd met someone when she was on jury duty who exemplified the worst of who she used to be. In her words, "This lady reeked of negativity, and I didn't want to be anything like her."

BE AWARE OF WHAT YOU TELL YOURSELF

For years I have witnessed clients get in the way of their own success because of how they think. It is no secret that we are constantly in conversation with ourselves, and if that inner dialogue isn't positive, it can be extremely discouraging. Knowing this, I have helped many people become more aware of what they are thinking, so that each time they catch themselves entering into negative self-talk, they can immediately come up with at least 10 positive thoughts to counteract each negative. We really need to be aware of what we are telling ourselves and be sure that our internal dialogue is supportive of our motivation and our goals. I tell my clients that they need to remember the three Ps:

Positive

Present

Personalized

We must be as aware of how we talk to ourselves as we are of the way we talk to others. Speak in positive terms; speak *as if* what you want were happening now, and be certain that what you focus on is specific to you.

To help you implement the three Ps, consider the following tips:

1. Repeat to yourself several times throughout the day what it is you want, but do it in a way that assumes it's already happened. For example, you might say, "I am reducing my waistline daily." Or, "I am constantly and consistently giving myself every opportunity to lose weight." Remember, all your positive statements are to be in the present, not in the future. As you affirm the statement to yourself, you are internalizing it so that your mind absorbs and embraces it as a command.

2. Use positive words when speaking and thinking. Positive words encourage and create positive emotions. What you say out loud is a manifestation of the way you think. At first, using positive words may take a lot of conscious effort, but soon it becomes a habit, and you'll find yourself feeling optimistic and upbeat instead of falling prey to negative thoughts when faced with moments of concern or challenge.

3. Create mental pictures of where you want to be. Doing so will fuel the achievement of what you'd like to see. If you can create a mental image of your future self and affirm with your words what you are achieving, you will significantly increase your positive outlook and your ability to bring your goals to fruition.

4. The more emotions you can evoke when making your positive statements, the greater their impact will be. So, instead of saying simply, "I am eating the right foods and losing weight," you might say, "I appreciate being able to eat real food and lose weight." By attaching a feeling of appreciation to what you are accomplishing, you will instantly boost positive feelings about yourself.

5. You cannot make positive statements too frequently. I recommend writing your statements on an index card that you keep by your bed, so that you can read your statements just before you go to sleep and as soon as you wake up. Also keep cards bearing your statements in your pocket, in your car, on your desk—wherever they will remind you to repeat them throughout the day.

HOW OFTEN DO YOU LIE TO YOURSELF?

There is real power in positive self-talk, but it's essential that when you make these positive statements you truly believe them and that you don't lie to yourself.

Let's say I've promised my daughter that we're going to leave for the zoo in 10 minutes. If we don't leave for 20 minutes, she may forgive me this one lapse, but if I do that often enough, she'll start to believe that when I say 10 minutes I really mean 20 minutes. So how does that relate to what you tell yourself? Well, the more you lie, the more comfortable you get with lying. It's a slippery slope. Then, if you tell yourself you're going to go to the gym and do 30 minutes of cardio, you might decide after 20 minutes that you've had a good workout and there are other things you need to do, so you're going to leave. You've lied to yourself, and you're okay with that. Now let's say you've told yourself you're ready to do what this book says; this is the last time you're going to have to lose weight because this time you're going to keep it off. If you've been lying in every other area of your life, you know you've just told yourself another lie, and you won't be motivated to follow through.

Once you've begun to focus on the positive, you need to make sure that you honor what you say to yourself. Lying to yourself is the surest way to kill your motivation. One lie leads to another, and before you know it, you'll be back to square one and have to start all over again. What will keep you moving forward is to tell yourself the truth, do what you say, and focus on the process.

BECOME OKAY WITH BEING PATIENT

Weight loss, like most things that are worth achieving, is a process, and it may take longer than you'd like. As a society, however, we're not very comfortable with the concept of patience. We want it now, whatever it is, and if we don't get it within the time frame we've predetermined, we tend to get frustrated and quit. That need for instant gratification can cause us to set unrealistic goals, which is just another way of lying to ourselves, which leads to the loss of motivation. One of the keys to achieving a diet-free life is to relearn the power of patience.

One woman who had started following the process in this book told me she was upset because it wasn't working. In the first 7 days she was down 1 pound. At the end of the next 7 days she was down a total of 3 pounds, and at the 21-day mark she'd lost 5 pounds. When I asked her why she was upset, she said, "Because I've lost only five pounds and you said I could lose seven in the first seven days. Plus, on all the other diets I've been on I lost much more than that in the first three weeks. Your method doesn't work."

I confess that I really wanted to laugh at that. Had she even heard what she'd just said? If "all the other diets" she'd been on were so great, why was she now using my way to lose weight? But I didn't laugh. Instead I said, "I'm sorry, but you can't compare my approach to any of those other diets. They were all negative. They were about deprivation. This time you lost five pounds *eating*. You weren't deprived, you weren't hungry, and you ate only food you liked. You ate breakfast, you snacked, you went to lunch, you snacked again, and you ate dinner. You're still eating many of the same foods that caused you to gain weight in the past, only now you're eating them the right way, so that those same foods are causing you to *lose* weight."

As I was saying all this to her, I saw the light of understanding come on in her eyes. She had set an unrealistic goal by lying to herself about her previous diets, and when she didn't reach that goal, she temporarily lost her motivation.

I had to get right up in her face and tell it like it was so that she would be able to keep it real.

What's real is being able to delay gratification, and what gets most dieters into trouble in the first place is not being able to do that. Being greedy, wanting it all, and wanting it now are what have allowed the supersize world to take advantage of so many of us.

The take-home lesson for this lady was that we are all different, and although some people do drop 7 pounds in 7 days, some lose less during their first 7 days using the Diet-Free Living ideas. Usually, the heavier you are, the more weight you can expect to lose in the first 7 days and thereafter. Nonetheless, you—like this woman and everyone else—can drop pounds and shed inches.

Because our metabolisms operate at different speeds, weight loss is achieved at different rates. Sometimes the weight comes off slower because of medications or because of years spent yo-yo dieting. The good news, however, is that as you get to know your body and how it responds to food and fitness, you'll be able to tweak your way of eating and exercising so that you speed up the process and learn how to keep the weight off.

IT'S ALL ABOUT YOU

When I told you about the three Ps, I said that you needed to keep it personal—that is, about you specifically. But most of us have been taught that it's selfish to put ourselves first, so if we make weight loss about us, we think our motivation is selfish.

Amy G. is a client who was having a problem sticking to her intention of getting to the gym three times a week because she worried that it would be taking time away from her children. She said that when she left work, even though she intended to get in a workout, she started thinking that she really ought to go home to her kids. I asked her how she felt when she put her own needs on the back burner by going home to her kids. "Horrible," she said. "Because I went another day without doing what I said I would." I asked her to think how she would feel if she went to the gym and *then* went home to the kids. Of course, her response was positive. I went on to assure her that taking care of herself is really the best thing for the kids *and* for her. This was Amy's aha moment, when she understood that by setting aside her own needs for what she thought was her children's welfare, she'd actually been cheating both herself and them. Doing what's best for everyone is the best motivation.

In another instance, Florence, who was attending one of my presentations, said that although she felt she was motivated, she was stuck. She wanted to lose weight and didn't know why she wasn't doing what she knew she wanted to do. We talked for a while about what might be stopping her, and she finally admitted that she was afraid that if she lost weight, she'd also lose her husband. It wasn't the first time I'd heard that notion. Sometimes if a woman loses weight, becomes more confident, and starts to dress differently, her partner may fear that he's losing control of the situation (and of her). He didn't marry a lean and confident woman, so "when she gets down, he may not be around."

Florence wasn't being foolish, and her fears weren't baseless, but I did tell her that if she knew in her heart of hearts that losing weight was what *she* wanted and needed, she had to do it for *herself*. If you neglect what you know is best for you to keep someone else happy, you're neither living your best life nor giving the best of who you are to others. If you're afraid to lose weight because it might upset someone else, what does that say about your self-esteem?

I gave Florence a homework assignment that day. I told her to keep working on her perception of her own worth, which removed this obstacle in her path to wellness.

For once in your life, you really do need to put yourself first. If you're looking for motivation to do that, tell yourself that by becoming your best, you'll also be giving the best of yourself to those you love and care for.

KEEP TOSSING FUEL ON YOUR MOTIVATIONAL FIRE

I can't say that every moment from now on is going to be easy. Some of what you'll be experiencing may negate what you believed in the past; some strategies won't work the way you thought they would. There's going to be a learning curve, as there is whenever you do something new. To keep yourself motivated, it can be extremely powerful to immerse yourself in stories about other people who have struggled and come out on top. Watch documentaries on television, listen to motivational CDs, and read uplifting biographies. There's always a story behind the glory, and you can fuel your own motivation by learning about other people who faced challenges and adversity but had the tenacity to keep going.

When I meet people who have lost weight, I applaud them, but I'm more interested in the challenges—the process that allowed them to prevail. Unfortunately, however, it's not uncommon for us to focus on what has been accomplished rather than on the process that led to that accomplishment. Take Walt Disney, for example. The man who is now known for his countless innovations was once fired by a newspaper editor for lack of ideas. He also went bankrupt more than once before achieving financial success. Babe Ruth, who held the record for hitting the most home runs, also had the record for the most strikeouts. Talk about nothing ventured, nothing gained! The lives of Disney and Ruth remind us of the importance of persistence and going for it each time you're up at bat.

Their stories make you better appreciate the fact that experiencing setbacks is just a part of the process that leads to achieving great things. One of my favorite sayings is "A setback is nothing but a setup for a comeback." Say this out loud and notice how good you feel. It's also a great mantra to repeat to yourself when you get off track. When you say those words out loud to yourself, you immediately begin to refocus on how you're going to move forward. Hear me now: A setback is a setup for a comeback. Who doesn't like a comeback?

Finally, these stories—and so many others—remind us to never give up and to trust that whatever happens has a purpose; we just need to take the time to figure it out. No matter how positive or negative an experience may seem, be thankful for your ability to be present and appreciate the moment.

There are no failures, only lessons! I urge you to keep this motto in mind as you start your journey toward fat loss and fitness. In Chapter 9, you will find a day-by-day calendar of mental exercises designed to help you make over your mindset so that living diet-free becomes your way of life.

3

Gain New Knowledge About Nutrition

You may be highly motivated, with a clear, realistic goal in mind, but if you don't know what to do to achieve that goal, it won't matter how motivated you are. And if you don't understand *why* you're doing what you do, you'll be much less likely to remain committed long enough to achieve success. If you're going to be diet-free, you need the knowledge that will continue to fuel your intention. So, now is the time to educate yourself about nutrition.

Nearly everyone is familiar with the three basic food sources (macronutrients): protein, fat, and carbohydrates. But you may not know, or may have been misinformed about, how they work in combination with one another and, most important of all, how they affect your blood sugar levels, your hunger, and your body's inclination to either gain or lose fat. Here's what you need to know about each of these major nutrients.

PROTEIN: THE FIRST COMPONENT OF MAXIMIZING FAT LOSS

Anything that ever had feet, fins, or wings, anything that ever walked, swam, or flew, is a protein. And if it's derived from something that walked, swam, or flew, such as chicken eggs, it's likely to be a protein source. Some vegetable products, such as tofu, tempeh, and soybeans, are good protein sources. (Please refer to Chapter 8 if you're a vegetarian or a vegan.)

Any food that is higher in protein than in carbohydrates or fat content is a protein source. So, for example, if you choose to eat a yogurt that is higher in carbs than either protein or fat, it's a carb, not a protein source. If you choose a yogurt that is higher in protein than carbs or fat, it's a protein source. So be sure to read the nutrition labels on packaged foods and learn to differentiate what makes a protein, carb, or fat source.

As you begin to eat in a way that maximizes fat loss, you will be making sure that you get an adequate amount of protein at every meal.

WE NEED FAT, JUST NOT TOO MUCH

We all need fat to maintain cellular integrity and for other essential biological functions, but we get all the fat we need from other foods, so we never actually have to *add* fat to a meal. I will tell you that eating some fat with your carbohydrates can help keep your blood sugar from spiking, but there are ways to accomplish the same thing that don't involve consuming fat calories.

And even though I'm not going to ask you to count calories, that doesn't mean calories don't count. Just keep in mind that 1 gram of fat has twice as many calories as 1 gram of either protein or carbohydrate.

CARBOHYDRATES: THE KEY TO DIET-FREE FAT LOSS

To live diet-free, you need to understand the relationship between carbohydrates and fat loss. Taking control of your carbs is the key to keeping your blood sugar level so that your body is burning fat as quickly as possible. With diet-free living, there are no bad carbs—there are only wrong and right ways to eat them. The wrong way causes you to gain unwanted body fat; the right way helps you lose it. The right way means:

- eating proteins and carbs in the right combinations
- eating at the right intervals

- eating the right-size portions

To understand *why* these three factors are so important, you need to know *how* the foods you eat have an impact on what's going on in your body.

Insulin and Blood Sugar Levels

Insulin is a hormone produced by the pancreas that regulates the level of glucose (sugar) in the blood. The human body requires a steady amount of glucose throughout the day for energy, and that glucose comes from the foods—specifically the carbohydrates—we eat. I call insulin the "fat-storing hormone" because it is insulin that triggers the removal of glucose from our blood for storage in our liver, muscles, cells, and adipose (fat) tissue. What people with diabetes have known for some time is that if you consume too many carbohydrates at one time, you can flood your blood with sugar, which then increases the amount of insulin in your blood and the amount of sugar that is likely to get stored as fat.

Here's what happens: most carbohydrates you eat are metabolized as glucose (sugar) in your body. When your body senses that there is glucose in your bloodstream, it triggers the release of insulin from your pancreas. The insulin then removes the glucose from the blood. Some of that glucose is burned as fuel to support all your bodily functions, and the rest is converted to glycogen (the storage form of glucose) and stored in the liver and muscles. But if there's more glucose in your blood than you can store in your liver and muscles or need to burn as fuel, what's left over circulates in your blood (triglycerides) or gets stored as fat. When that happens, I call it a food flood. By keeping your level of blood sugar from fluctuating to extremes, you prevent those spikes in glucose levels that result in the release of insulin and, therefore, more fat storage.

Q There's a weight loss program that recommends no more than 15 grams of sugar a day. What do you think about that?—Stacey B. (Jerseyville, IL)

A I don't recommend any program that would restrict daily carbs or sugar to no more than 15 grams. My goal is to put an end to the notion that we have to restrict or deprive ourselves of things like sugar and carbohydrates. Our body and brain's primary source of fuel is carbs. We maximize fat burning when we are eating carbs. If anything, make sure you are getting at least 100 grams of carbs, in the right combinations, as part of your daily intake of food.

The Effects of Glucagon

So if carbs trigger insulin, which in turn can result in fat storage, why not simply cut out carbs completely, which was the basis for the Atkins diet? The answer to that lies with another hormone: glucagon.

If your blood sugar drops too low because you're not eating enough carbs or because you're not eating often enough, your body triggers the release of glucagon, another hormone secreted by the pancreas that is closely related to insulin. The glucagon then signals the liver and muscles to convert stored glycogen back into glucose and recirculate it into your bloodstream.

So let's say you're busy working on some kind of project and you forget to eat. At some point you start to feel ravenous, so you tell yourself you'll just finish what you're doing and then you'll get something to eat. You may notice that after a while, you don't feel hungry anymore. That's because your low blood sugar has triggered the release of glucagon, your liver has converted glycogen back into glucose, and you now have glucose in your bloodstream again. Because there's glucose in the blood, your body releases more insulin, and the vicious circle of rising and falling blood sugar levels, fat burning and fat storing, is set into motion.

Therefore, you do need to eat carbs, and you need to eat them often enough to prevent your blood sugar from falling too low. Carbohydrates are the primary source of fuel for your brain and your body, so carbs are your friend, not your enemy. And there are no carbs that are off-limits. You just need to eat them in the right combinations and portion sizes to satisfy your body and brain without spiking your blood sugar levels, so that you are able to maximize fat loss. That's exactly what I'm going to teach you how to do.

Beyond the Glycemic Index

When we hear the word *carbs* these days, we tend to think about the glycemic index, which is largely responsible for carbs having gotten such a bad rap.

Created in 1981 by David Jenkins and his associates at the University of Toronto, the glycemic index was designed as a method of ranking the speed with which various carbohydrates elevate blood sugar levels. Sugar (pure glucose) was ranked 100, and every other carb was given a ranking relative to that. These rankings, however, are based on 50 grams of carbohydrate in a single food. They do not consider the nutrition value of the food, nor do they take into account how much of the food we generally consume in one meal, the way the food is prepared, how ripe it is (if it's a fruit or vegetable), or what other foods we might be eating with it, all of which significantly impact how quickly that food will be metabolized into glucose and, therefore, raise blood sugar levels.

Here's an example that always seems to surprise my clients. A baked potato is rated 93 (at the high end of high) on the glycemic index, whereas potato chips are rated 55 (which is actually at the low end of medium). How can that be, and does it mean you should give up baked potatoes and start eating potato chips instead? Obviously not, since a baked potato is rich in nutrients, and chips are not. The reason for the discrepancy is that potato chips contain fat, and fat slows down the rate at which carbohydrates are metabolized. The good news is that if you put a tablespoon of butter or a tablespoon of fat-rich sour cream on your baked potato, it will slow down the rate at which it turns into glucose. So yes, having butter on your baked potato is actually a *good* thing, so long as you don't overdo it.

But you don't *have* to add butter or sour cream to your potato. Nor do you have to be concerned with the potato's being rated 93 on the glycemic index. Why? Because, as I'll be explaining, when you're eating a fist-size potato with a protein (fish, chicken, steak, turkey) and another carb that's metabolized more slowly (broccoli, beans, asparagus), you slow down the impact the potato could have on your blood sugar. So, as you will soon get to experience for yourself, when you eat your carbs in the right combinations and portions, and when you snack at specific intervals to be sure that you are satiated and that your blood sugar levels don't fluctuate too much, you will automatically be burning fat.

In another of my favorite examples, changing the fruit you put on your morning bowl of oatmeal, cream of wheat, or grits can make the difference between adding or shedding inches. When you eat your cereal with a sliced banana, you're certainly eating good-quality food, but you're also likely to be consuming too many carbohydrates in a single meal. Replace the banana with blueberries or strawberries and add a protein (such as eggs, protein powder, or sausage) to your meal, and you are more likely to keep your blood sugar levels in a place that maximizes your body's ability to burn fat instead of storing it.

Just making small adjustments like these to the way you combine foods produces significant results.

BUT THERE'S MORE: LEPTIN AND GHRELIN

Although scientists are still in the process of determining the mechanism by which it works, leptin is a hormone secreted by fat tissue that signals the brain that we're full. What researchers have found is that obese people appear to be unresponsive to leptin, meaning that their brains are resistant to the signals it sends; therefore, they don't know when they're full.

Ghrelin (pronounced *GREH-lin*), on the other hand, is the hormone produced in the stomach and the pancreas that lets us know we're hungry. Ghrelin levels increase before meals and decrease after meals.

It's when those ghrelin levels are too high that we become ravenous, and we don't want that to happen because we don't want to trigger the conversion of glycogen into glucose and spike our blood sugar, and also because it's when we're ravenous that we're most likely to make unhealthy, waistline-expanding food choices. To avoid those pitfalls, you're going to be eating every two to three hours from the time you wake up in the morning until an hour before you go to bed. That means you'll be eating breakfast within 30 to 60 minutes of when you wake up; you'll be having a snack in the morning, then another meal at lunch, a snack in the afternoon, followed by dinner, and, depending when you eat your dinner and when you go to bed, perhaps another snack in the evening.

If that sounds too rigid to you, don't be discouraged, because on days when you're not able to eat and snack at these specific intervals, it's okay (although not ideal) to snack when you would normally eat lunch, and then eat lunch when you'd normally be having your afternoon snack. The key is to eat either a meal or a snack every two to three hours.

This may sound like a lot of eating, but it's not, so long as you stick to the portions I recommend for the foods you choose to eat. Remember, I said you'd be able to eat real food, but please understand—calories still count, and if you take in more calories than your body can metabolize and burn, no matter what you eat you're most likely going to gain weight.

The National Research Council provides a rough estimate of people's daily calorie needs based on how active they are. They estimate that a 140-pound woman who is relatively sedentary should consume about 1900 calories. For a relatively sedentary 175-pound man, the recommendation is 2400 calories per day.

I recommend that in order to lose weight, women should stick to 1200 to 1800 calories daily, and men to 1500 to 2300 calories daily. Based on the National Research Council guidelines, that would be a reduction of 700 calories per day for the average 140-pound woman, which would equate to losing 1 pound every 5 days. For the average man, the reduction would be 900 calories, or 1 pound every 4 days. The more you weigh and the bigger the calorie deficit, the more weight you will lose. And that's not including the extra calories you would burn if you also chose to exercise. However, you also don't want to go below those recommendations, because eating fewer than 1200 or 1500 calories could cause your metabolism to slow or result in your losing muscle rather than fat.

Sharon M. was on a weight-watching program that required her to count every calorie and stick to a very strict eating regimen. She said that despite the restrictions, she didn't feel deprived, and she was adamant that her way of "dieting" worked. She had lost more than 60 pounds and kept 30 of those pounds off for more than 2 years. Well, when Sharon heard me speak about the potential consequences of eating fewer than 1200 calories, she questioned me. So I invited her to come to my clinic and have a body composition analysis conducted. She accepted, and after she'd lost another 10 pounds on her program, I asked her to return so that we could take a closer look at what type of weight she had lost. Unfortunately, and much to her surprise, she had lost 8 pounds of lean body mass and only 2 pounds of fat.

That wake-up call caused Sharon to shift her mindset in regard to weight loss. She followed my advice, adding a balanced breakfast and more carbs to her daily nutrition, and as a result, she gained 10 pounds of lean body mass and lost 20 pounds of fat.

IN A STUDY reported in the *American Journal of Epidemiology* in 2003, researchers found that people who skipped breakfast were 4.5 times more likely to be overweight than those who ate breakfast regularly. In addition, researchers at Virginia Commonwealth University in Richmond found that people wanting to lose weight whose breakfast contained both protein and carbs lost four times more than those on a low-carb plan.

Eating breakfast means that you won't be starving when lunchtime rolls around, and therefore, you won't be tempted to eat too much. But it's also important to eat within 30 to 60 minutes of waking up because you have, in effect, been fasting all the while you were asleep, which means that your metabolism has slowed down. That's not a bad thing because it gives your metabolism time to rejuvenate. But then you need to eat breakfast to get it revved up again, and the sooner you do that the sooner you'll start burning more fat.

If you exercise within 30 to 60 minutes of waking up, you don't have to eat breakfast before you work out, but you should eat within 30 to 60 minutes after you finish. If you are diabetic or experience low blood sugar, I recommend you eat either a snack or breakfast before your morning exercise. I'll be giving you more information about the timing of food and exercise in Chapter 7.

FAST AND SLOW CARBS: THE KEY TO PROPER FOOD COMBINING

Even though you may be eating healthful foods right now, you may not be eating them in a way that keeps your blood sugar from fluctuating too low or too high. The cornerstone of my approach to shedding inches and dropping body fat is both to understand the proprietary formula I use to categorize carbs and to create a fat-burning meal that properly combines the macronutrients protein, carbs, and fat in appropriate portion sizes.

Fast carbs are those that raise your blood sugar relatively quickly when compared to slow carbs.

Slow carbs are those you metabolize more slowly and that are usually higher in fiber and protein and relatively lower in calories than fast carbs.

Fast carbs aren't necessarily bad, so long as you eat them in the portions and combinations I recommend. No single portion of food or meal should contain more than 45 grams of carbohydrates for women or 50 grams for men after you've subtracted the total grams of fiber. But just as you won't have to count calories, you won't have to weigh everything you eat, so long as you stick to the portion sizes I recommend. In Chapter 6 you'll find lists of fast and slow carbs as well as proteins, fats, and condiments, along with their proper portion sizes.

▶ Making Carbs Your Friend

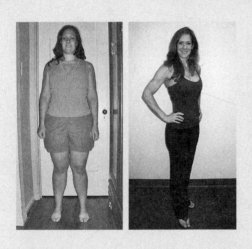

WHEN TWYLA M. joined my program and put my formula into practice, she got off to a great start: Within 21 days, she was down 13 pounds. Twyla was adamant about making sure she continued to eat carbs, but in the right way, of course, combining her fast carbs with protein and slow carbs. She wanted to make sure that as she shed the inches and dropped the pounds, it was not just a fad approach or something she couldn't sustain. She lost on average 2 pounds a week, going from 179 to 129 in 6 months. Then, after continuing to live diet-free, Twyla shifted gears and focused more on her body fat percentage. At 179 pounds, she was 34 percent. At 129, she was 24 percent. Today, after keeping the weight off for 2 years, Twyla is down to 119 pounds and 18 percent body fat.

Now that you know what you're going to be eating and why it works, it's time to figure out where you are now in terms of fat and fitness so that you can track your progress as you move toward your weight and fitness goals.

▶ Carbs and Fiber

MOST CARBS CONTAIN some fiber, but slow carbs tend to contain more fiber than fast carbs do. And when you're eating carbs, the good news is that you get to deduct the number of fiber grams from the total number of carb grams because fiber is not digestible and therefore doesn't add calories to your food. Better yet, fiber helps slow the conversion of carbs into blood sugar, thus reducing the impact sugar has on your blood.

So, if you're eating a carb that comes in a package with a label and you need to know how many grams are in a portion, subtract the fiber grams from the total number of carb grams to arrive at the number of grams you'll be consuming.

4

Where Are You Now?

You need to assess exactly where you're starting from so that you will be able to make the necessary changes and chart your progress. These are the same steps I ask each of my clients to take before they begin any weight loss program.

Before you go any further, buy yourself a notebook or journal. (Or go to my website at www.dietfreelife.com to learn about the 8 Week Fat Loss Planner for tracking food, fitness, and mood.) You'll be using your notebook or journal to keep track of your progress and to complete the 21-Day Mindset Makeover in Chapter 9. In addition, it will be extremely helpful to keep a record of everything you eat along with the time you consume it and how you feel (your mood) when you eat it. In fact, according to a study from Kaiser Permanente Center for Health Research—one of the largest and longest-running weight loss maintenance trials ever conducted—people who keep daily food records lose twice as much weight as those who do not keep records.

So, let's get started.

TAKE A PHOTO

You know what you look like, but as you start to look different, which you will, it's easy to forget what you looked like before. Our brain is great at forgetting what we'd rather not remember, but it's important that you *do* remember so that you can see for yourself how much progress you're making.

You could ask a close friend or family member to snap your photo, but most people would rather not do that. It's okay; you don't have to. With the technology available these days, it's easy to do it yourself.

Use a digital camera—I'm sure you can borrow one if you don't already own one. Set it up on a tripod or on a table or countertop about 3 feet off the ground and use the self-timer function. Step back far enough so that your entire body, from head to toe, appears in the photo (if you're doing this yourself, it may take a couple attempts before you get it just right), and stand against a plain background wearing contrasting clothing that reveals the "true you." If you're doing this in the privacy of your own home, that could be your underwear, a bathing suit, shorts, and, if you're a woman, a sports bra. You'll be wearing these same clothes again at the end of 7 days, when you assess your progress. Snap yourself from the front, side, and rear. Print your pictures and tuck them away in your journal.

TAKE YOUR MEASUREMENTS

Again, you need to do this so that you'll be able to chart your progress.

Using a cloth tape measure, take 14 measurements:

    1. Widest part of your neck

    2. Widest part of your chest

3 & 4. Widest part of your right and left upper arms

5 & 6. Widest part of your right and left forearms

7 & 8. Right and left wrists

    9. Waist (men: 1 inch below the navel; women: 1 inch above the navel)

  10. Widest part of your hips

11 & 12. Widest part of your right and left thighs

13 & 14. Widest part of your right and left calves

Be sure you remain relaxed while you're doing this. Don't tense your muscles; don't suck in your stomach. Be honest!

The reason it's so important to have these measurements is that you're going to be changing your body composition while you're losing weight. You're going to be dropping fat and gaining lean muscle tissue, and 1 pound of fat takes up six times more space in your body than 1 pound of muscle. Sometimes, in fact, you'll be dropping fat and gaining lean muscle tissue even when your scale weight stays the same, so you'll be losing inches even when you're not losing pounds. The pounds will come off, however; don't worry about that, because the more muscle you have, the faster you'll burn fat.

Now, record your measurements in your journal.

DETERMINE YOUR CURRENT PERCENTAGE OF BODY FAT

Fortunately, we now have a very easy way to determine your percentage of body fat: an impedance machine, or a scale that measures both your weight and your percentage of body fat. Some models even provide an estimate of how hydrated you are. The one I use is the Tanita scale, which is available from a variety of stores, including Walmart, Target, and Bed Bath & Beyond, as well as online from www.dietfreelife.com, www.amazon.com, and others. If you don't have one of these scales and can't afford to buy one, you can go to almost any health club, spa, or community center and get tested free of charge or for a nominal fee. My only caveat is that if you're using a scale at one of these locations, be sure that you continue to use the same one to monitor your progress. Different scales may be calibrated slightly differently, and if you go from one to another, you won't be getting an accurate picture of your progress.

There are other methods for measuring your body composition, but they may not be as convenient. For instance, the gold standard for determining body fat percentage is underwater testing (in a hydrostatic tank). While undoubtedly the most accurate, it is not always easily accessible.

If you can't get access to a hydrostatic tank or one of the impedance machines, use a cloth tape measure to keep track of the inches you lose in addition to monitoring your total body weight on a traditional scale. Don't rely solely on a traditional scale for determining whether you are making progress. Whatever method you choose to measure your progress, continue to use the same method as you go forward.

NOW DETERMINE YOUR FAT WEIGHT

Once you know your percentage of body fat, there's an easy formula for determining your fat weight. Just multiply your total weight by your percentage of body fat.

Total weight × percentage of body fat = fat weight

So if, for example, your total weight is 180 pounds and your percentage of body fat is 0.37, your fat weight is 66.60 pounds and your lean body weight is 113.40.

Now, write those numbers in your journal. You'll be using them to help determine where you want to be: your goal weight and percentage of body fat.

WHAT'S HOLDING YOU BACK?

Now that you've gotten up close and personal with your appearance, it's time to get better acquainted with your mind, specifically the obstacles you perceive to be preventing you from achieving the success you want. We're all very good at thinking of reasons why we *can't* do something, but the point here is to come up with strategies for overcoming those obstacles. The great general Sun Tzu wrote in *Art of War*, "If you know the enemy and know yourself, you need not fear the result of a hundred battles. If you know yourself but not the enemy, for every victory gained you will also suffer a defeat." Your obstacles, real or perceived, are the enemy, and you need to be consciously aware of them so that you can devise a plan to defeat them.

Take Gloria J., for example. Gloria was trying very hard to cut back on her consumption of fried foods, and when I asked her why she was having so much difficulty, she told me that she didn't get along very well with her mother-in-law, and every time she and her husband went to his mother's place for dinner, she served fried food. Not only that but she made a point of telling Gloria how hard she'd worked to cook the meal and urged her to try this or that. Gloria said that if she didn't eat the food, her mother-in-law would just have one more reason not to like her.

I agreed that she had a problem, but I explained that every problem had a solution, and she needed to come up with a contingency plan. What she needed to do was find a way to communicate with her mother-in-law that would shift the focus away from her not eating foods that are fried. I suggested that the next time they all sat down at the table and her mother-in-law urged her to taste something, Gloria might say, "I'm going to try that in a minute. It really looks delicious, but I want to finish what's already on my plate first. And by the way, how's your new job working out?" Or, "And tell me about your vacation; I hear it was terrific." In other words, she needed to *redirect* her mother-in-law's attention away from Gloria by getting her to talk about herself. Most people love to be invited to talk about themselves, and I assured Gloria the tactic would work. Sure enough, the next week when she came to see me she said that she'd managed to avoid the fried chicken by changing the subject to the beauty of her mother-in-law's rose garden, of which she was extremely proud.

Dennis V. had a different problem. He told me that for years his cousin had been coming to his house for breakfast every Sunday and bringing a big box of doughnuts. Dennis loved doughnuts and found them very hard to resist. He knew he'd never be able to "eat just one." But he also didn't want to hurt his cousin's feelings by asking him not to bring them.

I suggested to Dennis that he ask his cousin to bring bagels and cream cheese instead, and Dennis said he'd try but that it would be difficult because his cousin had been bringing the doughnuts for years, and it was a deeply ingrained habit, almost a ritual. So I asked Dennis what he'd do if his cousin brought the doughnuts even though he'd asked him not to, and he said he'd eat breakfast before his cousin arrived so that he'd be full and the doughnuts wouldn't be so tempting. Sure enough, the next Sunday rolled around and his cousin brought the bagels and cream cheese, but he *also* brought the doughnuts. Because Dennis had his contingency plan in place, however, he managed to resist the temptation.

So what are *your* obstacles? Get out your journal and take some time to really think about it as you write them down.

Here are some of the ones I hear most often:

I don't have time to plan meals. If this is your problem, purchase frozen entrees you can pop into the microwave so that you'll be able to enjoy a fat-burning meal in a matter of minutes. There are many good brands out there, so try a few and see which ones you like best.

I travel a lot and have a lot of business dinners. Whenever possible, go online and look at the menu options before going to the restaurant. When this isn't possible, keep an open mind, choose the best options available, and have a snack before you leave for dinner.

If I start cooking differently, my family isn't going to eat it. Cook the meal for yourself and taste-test it without expecting it to be a winner for your family. Ask everyone in the family to taste it and provide feedback you can use to determine whether it's going to become a staple for the family.

It's too complicated having to prepare all those different foods every day. Guess what, you don't have to prepare all those different foods every day. You're going to learn to eat foods that are readily available and already part of your environment in a way that helps your body optimize fat burning.

THE PROBLEM OF COMPETING INTENTIONS

Sometimes you may be dealing with two competing intentions, one that supports your goal and another that might put an obstacle in your path. The trick, then, is to find a way to satisfy both.

You might, for example, have an intention to stick to your fat loss plan, but you also want to go out to dinner with your girlfriends. If you want to do both, you need to have a strategy that will allow you to enjoy the evening without sabotaging your good intentions. Let's say that whenever you go out with the girls you go to the same restaurant, and you've always shared a big plate of chicken wings, which you all slather in ranch dressing and chase down with margaritas.

If you tell your friends you're not eating the wings because you're trying to eat healthier, you're clearly implying that what they're eating isn't healthy. Or if you order something else, which would be a change from the norm, you'd be calling attention to yourself, which would start them questioning you to figure out why.

One way to deal with the problem might be to do some research and figure out how many calories there are in those chicken wings. You might then decide to eat a couple of them as part of your meal. Or you might decide to have the wings and drink club soda instead of the margarita. Or perhaps you'll decide that seeing your friends is important enough for you to eat outside the parameters of the plan this one time and get back on track immediately after. Any one of those solutions would reconcile your competing intentions.

As I've said, and will be demonstrating in the chapters that follow, Fresh Start is about getting you up and running, and the 21-Day Mindset Makeover guides you to developing the mental attitude you need to make your lifestyle support your desire to be fit and healthy. The point is that you do need to have a plan as well as the mental tenacity to stick to the plan so that you won't be defeated by an obstacle you hadn't anticipated.

YOUR METABOLISM PROFILE

As the final step in the process of figuring out where you are, it's time to determine your current metabolism profile. Your answers to the following questions will let you know whether your body is currently more likely to store fat or burn it.

By completing this quiz, you will be better able to assess why your metabolism is perhaps not as fast as it once was and how you can make the small, easy adjustments that will speed it up and help you optimize your fat-burning potential. I have used this same quiz to help clients become aware of the control they have when it comes to food choices, portions eaten at a single time, and activity as it pertains to their fitness level.

Circle the one answer to each question that best applies to you. Your answers will help determine your Metabolism Score.

Personal Metabolism Profile Quiz

1. **How many times in your life have you dieted or enrolled in a program to lose weight?**
   A. I've never dieted
   B. Once
   C. Twice
   D. 3 to 6 times
   E. More than 6 times
   F. Too many times to count

2. **How often do you weigh yourself?**
   A. Only when I visit the doctor
   B. Rarely, if ever
   C. Once a week
   D. At least twice a week
   E. Once a day
   F. More than once a day

3. **Looking at your parents, do you think your body type is more likely to be:**
   A. Skinny but muscular
   B. Muscular
   C. Skinny
   D. Normal/Average
   E. Fat but muscular
   F. Fat

4. **How often do you eat breakfast?**
   A. Always
   B. 5 to 6 times a week
   C. 3 to 4 times a week
   D. 1 to 2 times a week
   E. Never

5. How often do you eat?
   A. 6 or more times a day
   B. 4 to 5 times a day
   C. 3 times a day
   D. Twice a day
   E. Once a day

6. What is your favorite type of food?
   A. Japanese
   B. Thai
   C. Mediterranean/Middle Eastern
   D. American
   E. Chinese
   F. Fast Food
   G. Hispanic
   H. Italian

7. Which of the following types of carbohydrates do you like most?
   A. Vegetables
   B. Fruit
   C. Cereal
   D. Bread
   E. Pizza
   F. Pasta
   G. Desserts

8. Which of the following proteins do you like most?
   A. Fish
   B. Turkey
   C. Chicken
   D. Tofu
   E. Pork
   F. Steak

9. **Which of the following condiments are you most likely to use for flavoring your foods?**
- **A.** Herbs and seasoning
- **B.** Mustard
- **C.** Sauces (BBQ, hot sauce)
- **D.** Salt
- **E.** Ketchup
- **F.** Cheese
- **G.** Butter
- **H.** Mayonnaise

10. **The first place you tend to gain weight is:**
- **A.** Evenly throughout your body
- **B.** In the face
- **C.** Upper body
- **D.** Lower body
- **E.** Midsection

11. **Which type of alcohol do you prefer?**
- **A.** I don't drink alcohol
- **B.** Wine
- **C.** Shots
- **D.** Mixed drinks
- **E.** Beer

12. **Which type of exercise do you prefer?**
- **A.** Lifting weights
- **B.** Playing sports
- **C.** Walking or hiking
- **D.** Performing cardio
- **E.** Participating in group exercise classes
- **F.** No exercise at all

13. On average, how many hours of sleep do you get each night?

A. More than 8 hours

B. 8 hours

C. 7 hours

D. 6 hours

E. Less than 5 hours

14. During a typical week, how often do you exercise?

A. 6 times a week

B. 4 to 5 times a week

C. 2 to 3 times a week

D. Whenever I can

E. Rarely, if ever

F. I don't exercise

15. How often do you have a bowel movement?

A. 3 or more times a day

B. Twice a day

C. Once a day

D. Every other day

E. 1 to 2 times a week

F. 1 to 3 times a month

16. On a typical day, how many hours do you go without eating something?

A. 2 hours

B. 3 hours

C. 4 hours

D. 5 to 6 hours

E. I only eat 1 or 2 meals a day

17. **When you eat a sandwich or a burger, what side dish do you include?**
- **A.** Nothing else
- **B.** Salad
- **C.** Fruit
- **D.** Chips
- **E.** Fries

18. **How many slices of bread do you usually eat in a day?**
- **A.** 1 slice
- **B.** 2 slices
- **C.** 3 slices
- **D.** I rarely eat bread
- **E.** 4 slices
- **F.** 5 or more slices

19. **When you snack, which of the following do you prefer to eat?**
- **A.** Fresh fruit
- **B.** Energy bar
- **C.** Cheese/nuts
- **D.** Something salty
- **E.** Candy/pastries/chocolate
- **F.** I rarely, if ever, snack

20. **Which of the following are you most likely to drink in the evening?**
- **A.** Water
- **B.** Tea
- **C.** Diet soda
- **D.** Fruit juice
- **E.** Alcohol
- **F.** Regular soda

Now Determine Your Score

Give yourself the following points for each answer you circled:

A. A = 5
B. B = 4
C. C/D = 3
D. E/F = 2
E. G/H = 1

My total is: _____45_____

What Your Score Means

85 and above. You scored high, which means that slight, simple changes to what you are already doing will significantly boost your metabolism in a way that brings about dramatic changes in your weight and body composition.

> **Example:** A simple change may be adding resistance training (lifting weights, strength training) to your fitness regimen to lower your body fat percentage and maximize fat loss.

75–84. Your metabolism is healthy, but you can boost it even more by changing some of the ingredients in the snacks and foods you are currently eating to help you quickly shift your body from being more likely to store fat to being more likely to burn it, and to tighten and tone your physique.

> **Example:** A simple change might be choosing products that don't have partially hydrogenated oils among the first four listed ingredients.

65–74. Learning how to combine the foods you are already eating and snacking the right way more often will maximize your metabolism and keep you from falling prey to the metabolic misfortune that results from continual shifts in your blood sugar levels.

> **Example:** A simple change would be to make sure you are not eating too many carbs in your meals and that your snacks aren't too high in calories but are high enough in carbs to prevent a drop in blood sugar.

0–65. Learning what to eat, when to eat it, and how much to eat is essential for increasing your metabolism and losing all the weight you want without ever feeling deprived.

Example: You will benefit most from a structured plan you can follow with ease and convenience.

What Your Answers Say About You

1. **How many times in your life have you dieted or enrolled in a program to lose weight?**
Yo-yo dieting often results in a slowed metabolism. Gaining weight and losing it only to gain it again throws your metabolism into a tizzy. No matter what your experience, however, you will benefit from embracing a lifestyle that supports a faster metabolism.

2. **How often do you weigh yourself?**
Weighing yourself often is usually an indication that you are too concerned with your scale weight. I recommend weighing yourself once a week at most on a scale that also gives your percentage of body fat.

3. **Looking at your parents, do you think your body type is more likely to be . . .**
Our body type may be, at least in part, inherited from our parents, but our taste, cultural eating habits, and lifestyle choices are also handed down from generation to generation. Although we can't control our genetics, we can change our eating habits and our lifestyle to maximize our metabolism and minimize our percentage of body fat.

4. **How often do you eat breakfast?**
Over the years, more than 70 percent of the clients who came to me had not made breakfast a regular habit. Not eating breakfast is a primary reason for having a slow metabolism. Eating breakfast regularly and in a timely manner is one of the easiest steps you can take to speed up your metabolism.

5. **How often do you eat?**
Going long periods of time without eating either a meal or a snack slows your metabolism. By eating every 2 to 3 hours, you speed up your metabolism.

6. What is your favorite type of food?

Although you can be lean and fit eating any type of food, people who primarily eat a traditional Japanese diet have been shown to have a quicker metabolism than those who follow a primarily Hispanic or Italian diet. In the following chapter, you will learn not only why most of the foods that are typically identified as Hispanic and Italian result in weight gain but also how to eat these same foods in a new way, so that you get a fresh start and begin to lose fat.

7. Which of the following types of carbohydrates do you like most?

Although you can be healthy eating any type of food, people who eat more vegetables tend to have a lower percentage of body fat and a faster metabolism than those who prefer breads, pasta, and desserts.

8. Which of the following proteins do you like most?

People who get the majority of their protein from leaner sources consume less saturated fat and are less likely to weigh down their metabolism.

9. Which of the following condiments are you most likely to use for flavoring your foods?

Higher-fat condiments are largely tied to a higher percentage of body fat and a sluggish metabolism.

10. The first place you tend to gain weight is . . .

While you can't control where you tend to gain weight, people with extra weight in the midsection tend to have a slower metabolism and may be at higher risk for health problems. Eating properly and exercising regularly are the two keys to increasing your metabolism and losing that midsection weight.

11. Which type of alcohol do you prefer?

Beer and mixed drinks are highest in calories and, therefore, most likely to cause you to gain weight.

12. Which type of exercise do you prefer?

A sedentary lifestyle correlates to a slow metabolism. The more active you are, the faster your metabolism.

13. On average, how many hours of sleep do you get each night?

Ideally, our metabolism benefits most when we get 7 to 8 hours of sleep a night. This optimal amount of sleep contributes to the repairing and rebuilding of our bodies and a quicker metabolism. A National Health and Nutrition Examination Survey found that people who get fewer than 4 hours of sleep a night are about 70 percent more likely to be overweight or obese than those who get 7 or 8 hours of sleep a night, those who get fewer than 5 hours are 50 percent more likely to be overweight, and those who get fewer than 6 hours are about 20 percent more likely to be overweight.

14. During a typical week, how often do you exercise?

The more active you are, the more likely it is that your metabolism will be working in high gear. Increasing activity of any kind will speed up your metabolism.

15. How often do you have a bowel movement?

Bowel movements are an indication of how quickly you metabolize your food. Regular eating along with regular bowel movements correlates with a well-functioning metabolism.

16. On a typical day, how many hours do you go without eating something?

Eating at the right intervals is a great way to use food to speed up your metabolism.

17. When you eat a sandwich or a burger, what side dish do you include?

Flooding your system with too many carbs (such as chips or fries with your burger on a bun) reduces the efficiency of your metabolism and positions your body to store fat instead of burn it.

18. How many slices of bread do you usually eat in a day?

I have found that clients who eat one to two slices of bread a day tend to have less body fat than those who eat more.

19. When you snack, which of the following do you prefer to eat?

In terms of maximizing your metabolism, eating something is always better than eating nothing. That said, however, snacks with lower levels of fat, salt, and refined sugar are more often correlated with a lower percentage of body fat.

20. **Which of the following are you most likely to drink in the evening?**
Water and tea contribute more than any other beverage to revving up your metabolism and helping you metabolize fat more efficiently. Make it your goal to consume a minimum of 8 to 12 (8-ounce) glasses of water daily to boost metabolism and optimize fat burning. And be sure to consume an additional 8-ounce glass of water for every 20 minutes of exercise. Also, if you are in a humid area, it is best to consume more water.

Look at your completed quiz and see which answers you scored lowest on. Those are the areas in which you will probably be making the greatest changes.

So, now that you know where you are mentally and physically, let's move on to figuring out where you want to be.

5

Where Do You Want to Be?

You may think you already know where you want to be, but I'll bet that, like many of my clients, the goal you now have in mind is based on incomplete or inaccurate information about what constitutes a healthy goal weight and/or body fat percentage.

Take Karen J., for example. When Karen first came to me, she was 72 years old and she'd been dieting since the age of 12—effectively for her entire life. As a kid, she'd go to the doctor, who weighed and measured her and said she needed to lose weight. Then, as a young adult, her doctor consulted the Metropolitan Life Insurance Company's Desirable Height and Weight Table for Men and Women, which was introduced in 1943 and revised slightly in 1983, and is based on statistics about people with the lowest mortality rates. According to the table, Karen was technically overweight.

In time, however, it became clear to many health and fitness professionals that standard charts and tables were not designed to take into account individual differences in body composition—bone density and amount of muscle, for instance—so the body mass index (BMI) became the new gold standard for determining whether a person is overweight, and it became Karen's new standard as well. The BMI was established in the mid-1800s by Adolphe Quetelet, a Belgian astronomer, mathematician, statistician, and sociologist (not a medical doctor). But the BMI, which is designed to determine a person's percentage of body fat based on his or her scale weight, doesn't take body composition into account any more than do the common height and weight charts. It doesn't adjust for bone density or lean muscle tissue, the weight of your organs, or the amount of water in your body.

When I explained to Karen the fallacies in the way she had been determining her goal weight and said that what was really important was her *body composition*—specifically her percentage of body fat as opposed to everything else—she found it very difficult to believe. I said that her real goal ought to be losing the fat and hanging on to as much of her lean body mass as possible, and even though she was still emotionally wedded to the number on the scale, she was willing to try it my way.

After 3 weeks, Karen had lost a total of 4 pounds, and she was discouraged because, as she told me, "I thought I was doing everything right." I assured her that she had, indeed, done everything right. And, sure enough, when we looked at the change in her body composition, she had lost 8 pounds of body fat and gained 4 pounds of lean body mass, which meant she had also increased her metabolism (the rate at which she was burning calories) because muscle tissue is significantly more metabolically active (that is, burns calories more efficiently) than fat. She knew she'd lost inches (15 inches in 21 days), but she was still looking to the scale for confirmation and gratification. All her life, people had been telling her it was the number on the scale that mattered, and I was the only person telling her something different. That was hard for Karen to accept, and it may be hard for you as well. That's why, again, I'm asking you to take it on faith and experience it for yourself so that you will ultimately come to believe it.

SHEDDING INCHES VERSUS DROPPING POUNDS

People who have dieted on and off tend to lose body weight more slowly when they begin living diet-free. What often happens is that they first shed inches, meaning that they get smaller, while they are boosting their metabolism. Their scale weight may not move as fast as they'd like, but as I keep saying, the goal shouldn't be just to lose scale weight but to lose inches and increase metabolism.

Keep in mind as you go forward that your ultimate goal is to get smaller and retain as much lean muscle tissue as possible while burning off fat. When it comes to weight loss, the winner is the one who sheds inches as opposed to merely dropping pounds. It's the fat weight that hinders our health and causes our clothes to feel tight and uncomfortable. It's the fat weight we pinch and hate. So everything I present in this book is about burning and releasing fat, not just weight.

WHY RETAINING LEAN BODY MASS IS IMPORTANT

Given my profession, people often come up to me at social events to tell me about the great diet they went on and how much weight they've lost. "Hey, Robert, I lost thirty pounds on this fabulous new diet!" My answer to that is, "That's great, but thirty pounds of what?" And the person is totally at a loss.

It's important to know where our weight loss is coming from because as we mature, it becomes more and more important to maintain our lean muscle tissue and bone density to optimize functionality. If you've ever seen a person who is seriously ill and in the hospital, you've probably noticed that he or she has lost a lot of weight and generally looks pale and gaunt. That's because that person has lost lean muscle tissue and is probably feeling as weak as he or she looks. If, on the other hand, you lose fat and gain lean muscle, you won't look sick and you won't be weak; you'll be looking healthy and vibrant, and you'll also increase your strength and energy. Therefore, people who measure their weight loss progress strictly by the number on the scale are doing themselves a big disservice.

Losing muscle, or what scientists call sarcopenia (pronounced *SAR-co-PEEN-yuh*), not only slows your metabolism so that you burn fewer calories but also causes more fat to be deposited in muscle cells, which is what we refer to as muscle marbling. (That's great for a steak but not for you!) In addition, less muscle means weaker bones and compromised balance. Again, all weight loss is not created equal, which is why I want you to know the difference between merely losing weight and losing fat. According to Ben Hurley, a professor of exercise physiology at the University of Maryland in College Park, women in their 40s and men in their 60s lose muscle strength at a rate of about 12 percent per decade. The good news is that no matter where you stand today, following the principles I outline in this book will lead to a dramatic improvement in your body composition.

Q I have been told that your body will break down muscle before fat if you do not have the right nutrition. Is this true? —Donald M. (Knoxville, TN)

A Your body is always burning fat. The primary reason that our bodies break down muscle is that we are not eating enough calories and/or carbohydrates or exercising in the right way. When your calorie or carbohydrate intake is too low, your body will turn to its carb storage areas, such as your liver and muscles, for energy. And when you don't use your muscles, you eventually lose them.

LOOKING LEAN AND WEIGHING MORE

If you knew what some of our leanest, fittest athletes actually weigh, the number would probably be much higher than you'd ever have guessed. Why? Think about this: A pound of feathers and a pound of lead both weigh a pound, but a pound of feathers takes up a lot more room than does a pound of lead. And the same is true of muscle and fat. A pound of fat takes up a lot more room in your body than does a pound of muscle, so when the ratio of muscle to fat changes for the better, even if you lost no weight at all, you still look a lot smaller because you lost inches.

Would you like to be smaller and wear a smaller size, or would you like to be the same size but weigh less? Fortunately, with all that you learn in this book, you can lose both inches and scale weight.

DETERMINE YOUR DESIRED PERCENTAGE OF BODY FAT AND YOUR GOAL WEIGHT

You've already determined your current fat weight, lean body weight, and percentage of body fat, so what you want to do now is figure out how much of that fat you want to lose. By focusing on the percentage of body fat you want to achieve, you are going to determine what a healthy body weight is for you.

Remember that you need to have some fat. In fact, as I've said, fat is essential for maintaining the integrity of your cell walls and other bodily functions. In addition, by nature, women have about 5 percent more body fat than men to maintain menstruation and a developing fetus. Also, women have more enzymes for storing fat and fewer enzymes for burning fat. Men have more lean muscle tissue and, therefore, less body fat.

To help you determine your desired percentage of body fat, I've provided a chart that is based on guidelines from the American Council on Exercise (ACE), the National Institutes of Health, and the World Health Organization as reported by the New York Obesity Research Center. These are the same guidelines we use at my clinic.

Female
General Body Fat Percentage Categories

AGE	HEALTH RISK*	ATHLETIC	HEALTHY**	OVER FAT	OBESE
18–39	Under 12%	13–20%	21–32%	33–38%	39%+
40–59	Under 12%	15–22%	23–33%	34–39%	40%+
60–99	Under 12%	17–23%	24–35%	36–41%	42%+

Male
General Body Fat Percentage Categories

AGE	HEALTH RISK*	ATHLETIC	HEALTHY**	OVER FAT	OBESE
18–39	Under 6%	6–13%	14–20%	21–24%	25%+
40–59	Under 6%	8–14%	15–22%	23–27%	28%+
60–99	Under 6%	12–20%	21–25%	26–29%	30%+

*When body fat percentage drops too low, you can be at risk for various health problems.

**Please note that "healthy" in this chart is used to indicate an average range and does not necessarily mean that if you have more or less body fat you are unhealthy.

Once you've decided on your desired percentage of body fat, you can go on to determine your goal weight. Remember that the goal is to lose fat while retaining as much lean muscle tissue as possible. Therefore, to determine your goal weight, you use the following formula.

1. Subtract your goal percentage of body fat from 100.
2. Divide your current lean body weight by that number to determine your goal weight.

So, for example, if you currently weigh 200 pounds and your current body fat percentage is 0.40, your total fat weight is 80 pounds and your total lean body weight is 120 pounds. Therefore, if you determine that your goal percentage of body fat is 0.25, you calculation would be as follows:

TOTAL	100
Goal body fat percent	0.25
Subtraction	0.75
120 divided by 0.75 =	160 pounds

This is what you would weigh if you got to your desired 25 percent body fat without losing any of your lean body mass.

REMEMBER, IT'S A PROCESS

Based on where you are now, you may think it's impossible to reach these goals. You may be so upset—amazed, horrified, surprised, disappointed, you name it—by your current weight and percentage of body fat that you're discouraged from moving forward. If so, just remember the ancient Chinese proverb, "A journey of one thousand miles begins with a single step." Your goal may seem far off, but with each percent or half percent of body fat you shed, you will be that much closer to your destination. Don't let the numbers stop you; keep repeating your positive statements to yourself and *believe* that you can change . . . because you can.

When my 46-year-old client Darla L., who weighed 313 pounds, hired me to coach her from 55 to 27 percent body fat, there were moments when her doubt almost made *me* doubt, but I knew it was possible. I just had to get her to believe it. Fortunately, in less than 6 months, Darla came to see the statement "I'm possible" hidden in the word *impossible*. Along the way, Darla would drop a half to a full percent of body fat only to see it come back, even though her total weight continued to go down. As confusing as that was, we kept our eye on the goal and continued to make adjustments until Darla weighed in at 156 pounds and 26.2 percent body fat.

You, too, may find that as you are losing weight, your percentage of body fat versus lean body mass will fluctuate, and in the chapters that follow, I'll provide you with the same troubleshooting tips I gave Darla, so that, in the end, you'll be losing a maximum of fat and gaining a maximum of lean muscle tissue.

Just keep telling yourself that it's a process, and make sure that what you want is achievable.

KEEP IT REAL

One thing people often ask me is if they're ever going to get back to the "fighting weight" they were at when they graduated high school. And my answer to that is, if you weighed 125 pounds when you graduated high school but you've been carrying 200 pounds for the last 20 years, your bones have become heavier, and you've also gained muscle (to support all that weight), so if you did get back to 125, you'd be giving up bone and muscle along with the fat, and you'd probably look as if you ought to be in the hospital. So you may not get back the exact body you had 20 years ago, but that's okay. You didn't want to go backward anyway, did you?

To keep it real, you have to know not only what is possible and what you want but also what you're willing to do to get it. In other words, you need to evaluate your own lifestyle. But if you think that you want to radically change your entire life, realistically that may not be feasible for you. So if someone tells me he or she wants to work out 6 days a week, I say, "Okay, but let's look at what you're life is really like. You work x number of hours a week, you pick up the kids, and most nights you also make dinner for the family. Really think it through and then tell me again how many times a week you can work out." The second answer is always different from the first. So let's say this person comes back and tells me it's going to be 3 days a week. I say, "Okay, let's plan on two." "But I told you I could do three!" "Okay then, if you do three, that's a bonus. But if you say two and you really do it, you'll start building confidence and you'll get better at following through. On the other hand, if you say three and do two, you'll be lying to yourself, and one lie is likely to lead to another. Sometimes less is best."

Do you drive a lot? Do you plan to eat out a lot? Sometimes people whose life requires that they spend a lot of time in their car go on a diet that requires them to prepare all their meals. Either they need to find a microwave on the road or they have to eat their meals cold. Pretty soon they have a collection of old plastic containers on the backseat of their car. They stick with it for a while, but it doesn't work over time because it doesn't fit in with the rest of their life.

My plan is different. If you know you eat lunch out every day, we're going to come up with a plan to support that. If you spend a lot of time in airplanes, we're going to plan for that. For the next 7 days, you're not going to drastically change anything.

WHAT ABOUT EXERCISE?

I've mentioned exercise a few times so far, but for the first 7 days you're living diet-free, you're not going to worry about that. If you've been totally sedentary, you don't have to suddenly start running (or even walking) 5 miles a day. If you've been doing some exercise, continue to do whatever it is you've been doing.

Ultimately, adding some exercise to your life is going to help you build lean muscle, and if you want to start that now, you can turn to Chapter 10 to get some tips on how to do it. But if you don't, you'll still see results at the end of the first week.

The only thing I ask is that you don't reduce or stop whatever exercise you *have* been doing because that may cause you to *lose* lean muscle and, therefore, slow your metabolism, at least in the short run. Even athletes who can't exercise due to sickness or injury lose some muscle tone. But it comes back very quickly as soon as they resume their exercise routine.

Now that you have all the information you need about where you are, where you want to be, and the science that supports the means to get you there, it's time to get going.

6

Start to Maximize Your Fat Loss

Although there are thousands of foods on this planet, I'm making it easy for you to eat common everyday real foods and still lose weight by providing a list of those most often eaten for breakfast, lunch, and dinner. They run the gamut from Italian to Mexican to Asian to soul food and take into account regional preferences of the east, west, north, and south. When you use the foods on these lists in the proper combinations and quantities, you will be maximizing your fat loss.

MAKE PROTEIN THE CENTERPIECE OF EVERY MEAL

To make sure that you are boosting your metabolism and maximizing fat loss, you'll be eating a minimum of 15 grams of protein at every meal. Protein promotes feelings of satiety and keeps you satisfied longer than carbohydrates alone do, in part because it takes longer to digest and also, when eaten with carbs, it slows down the rate at which you metabolize them. In addition, protein is essential for the healthy maintenance of your muscles, organs, skin, and nails. Many of your hormones are made up of protein, and protein is used in the manufacture of the red blood cells that carry oxygen throughout the body. Simply put, you cannot live without protein. Beyond that, however, your body burns more calories when digesting protein than it does when digesting fats or carbohydrates. Therefore, eating protein is an easy way to boost your metabolism.

When people are losing weight but most of the loss is coming from their lean body mass (rather than from fat), it's often because they aren't eating enough protein. If you're in that situation, the easy fix is to evaluate your daily protein intake and figure out a way to bump it up a little. One great tactic I've used with clients time and again is to replace one or two of their common snacks with something higher in protein, such as an energy bar, jerky, cottage cheese, or slices of deli meat.

Here's a list of the proteins and portion sizes you can choose from to make up your fat-burning meal.

Q When eating on the go or choosing a frozen entrée, is there a caloric range for what makes a fat-burning meal?—Kelley H. (Vancouver, BC)

A When you have your minimum protein and carbs, without having too many carbs, the caloric range of a fat-burning meal for women is 300 to 500 and for men, 400 to 600.

Lean Protein

For common lean proteins, the recommended portion size is 4 to 6 ounces for men and 3 to 5 ounces for women. This is generally a serving size of the area from the bottom of your palm to the first knuckle. If you're concerned about your ability to judge accurately from a visual cue, you can buy an inexpensive digital scale and weigh your portions for a while, until you become more confident.

- Eggs*
- Wild game (venison, bison, ostrich)
- Soy/tofu (all types)

---

*For men, a portion equals 2 whole eggs plus 2 egg whites or egg substitute. If you want to eat egg whites or substitute alone, the recommended portion size is 5 to 6 ounces (¾ cup). For women, a portion equals 1 whole egg plus 2 egg whites or substitute. If you want to eat egg whites or substitute alone, the recommended portion size is 3 to 4 ounces (½ cup). Note: 1 ounce egg white = 2 tablespoons, or ⅛ cup.

- Skinless chicken and turkey breast
- Lean fish and shellfish (Albacore tuna, halibut, tilapia, snapper, mahi mahi, shrimp, scallops)

Not-as-Lean Protein

For proteins that tend to be higher in fat than those already listed, the portion size is 4 ounces for men and 3 ounces for women. That would be a serving equal to the size of your palm.

- Steak (filet mignon, rib eye, sirloin, flank)
- Ground beef
- Ham
- Hot dogs
- Sausages*
- Bacon*
- Fatty fish (salmon, sardines, herring, lake trout)

▶ The Dairy Dilemma

MOST DAIRY IS a combination of protein and carbohydrates, and many dairy products are also loaded with fat. Check the label to see how many grams of each the product contains. Whichever is highest determines the category it's in. And that's true for all other packaged foods you buy.

FAST AND SLOW CARBOHYDRATES

As I explained in Chapter 3, one factor in keeping your blood sugar level even and, therefore, maximizing your metabolism and your fat loss is to eat

---

*The recommended portion size for sausage links and bacon is usually 2 links, 2 slices of Canadian, or 4 slices of cured because of the increased amount of fat calories in these foods.

carbohydrates in the proper combinations and the proper quantities—not to stop eating carbs altogether

For foods that aren't packaged or don't provide a calorie count, use the guidelines provided in the following charts.

▶ What's a Proper Portion?

COMMON FAST CARBS, such as breads and bagels, can vary greatly in size, so be sure to read the label and keep your portion to no more than 27.5 grams (or 110 calories) a slice. Although I'm not asking you to count all your calories, when you're buying packaged bread, it's a good idea to look at the nutritional breakdown on the label to be sure you aren't consuming more than 220 calories of bread in a single meal.

Fast Carbohydrates

FAST CARB	PORTION SIZE	
	Women	Men
Apple	1 medium	1 large
Bagel (3–4 inches in diameter)	1 whole	1 whole
Banana	1 medium	1 large
Beans (dried)	½ cup	⅔ cup
Bread (sliced)	2 slices	2 slices
Cantaloupe	2 cups	2½ cups
Cereal*	Follow serving size on box	
Corn kernels**	½ cup	⅔ cup
Corn tortilla (6 inches in diameter)	4	4
Couscous (pasta)	½ cup	⅔ cup
Cream of wheat (cooked)	1 cup	1¼ cup
English muffin	1	1
Flour tortilla (6 inches in diameter)	1	1
Grits (hominy, cooked)	1 cup	1¼ cup
Honeydew melon	2 cups	2½ cups

FAST CARB	PORTION SIZE	
	Women	Men
Macaroni and cheese	1 cup (4 ounces)	1¼ cups (5 ounces)
Milk (all types, except coconut)	1 cup	1 cup
Oatmeal (cooked)	1 cup	1¼ cup
Orange	1 medium	1 large
Pancakes (5 inches in diameter)	2	3
Pasta (cooked)	1 cup (4 ounces)	1¼ cups (5 ounces)
Peach	1 medium	1 large
Pear	1 medium	I large
Potato, baked	The size of your fist	
Quinoa	½ cup	⅔ cup
Rice (all kinds)	½ cup	⅔ cup
Squash (acorn, butternut, spaghetti)	1 cup (4 ounces)	1¼ cups (5 ounces)
Sweet potato (yam)	1 cup (4 ounces)	1¼ cups (5 ounces)
Waffles	2	2
Watermelon	2 cups	2½ cups

*When you combine a serving of cereal with 8 ounces (1 cup) of milk, you have a complete fat-burning meal. Even though both the cereal and the milk are fast carbs, when eaten together they provide enough protein and not too many carbs to create a fat-burning meal.

**Or 1 ear of corn on the cob.

Q I'm having trouble finding really good bread. I find breads that have whole wheat as the first ingredient, but then the second ingredient is usually enriched white flour. What bread do you eat?—Carly H. (Muncie, IN)

A If you want to avoid enriched wheat, go with a sourdough bread. It has white flour but no sugar, and because of the acidity in the bread, it converts to sugar in your blood more slowly than whole wheat does. Otherwise, keep looking; there are now many breads available that do not have any enriched wheat flour.

FAQ

Slow Carbohydrates

SLOW CARB	PORTION SIZE	
	Women	Men
Apricot	1 cup	1¼ cups
Artichoke hearts	½ cup	⅔ cup
Asparagus (cooked)	1 cup	1¼ cups
Beans (all types, except dried)	½ cup	⅔ cup
Beet greens	1 cup	1¼ cups
Beets	1 cup	1¼ cups
Bell pepper	1 cup	1¼ cups
Berries (strawberries, blueberries, raspberries)	1 cup	1¼ cups
Broccoli	1 cup	1¼ cups
Brussels sprouts	1 cup	1¼ cups
Carrots	1 cup	1¼ cups
Collard greens	1 cup	1¼ cups
Dandelion greens	1 cup	1¼ cups
Eggplant	1 cup	1¼ cups
Grapefruit (whole)	Medium	Large
Kale	1 cup	1¼ cups
Mushrooms (portobello and shitake)	1 cup	1¼ cups
Mustard greens	1 cup	1¼ cups
Peas (all types)	½ cup	⅔ cup
Summer squash (pattypan, pumpkin, yellow, zucchini)	1 cup	1¼ cups
Swiss chard	1 cup	1¼ cups
Tomatoes (all varieties)	1 cup (1 whole)	1¼ cups
Turnip greens	1 cup	1¼ cups

All of the following are eat-all-you-want raw vegetables, meaning that you can have as much as you want as part of your meal. When eaten raw, these vegetables are so low in calories and high in fiber that you can pack your plate with them and still maximize fat loss.

Diet-Free for Life

Cauliflower

Celery

Cucumbers

Mushrooms (button, crimini, and white)

Peppers (green and red)

Radishes

Raw leafy greens (arugula, bok choy, cabbage, endive, lettuce, radic-
chio, spinach, and watercress)

Sprouts

Q Eating and drinking healthier seems to cause me to have gas and
bloating. What do you recommend I do to keep this from happening?—Chris T. (Morrisdale, PA)

A It's likely that the added gas and feeling of being bloated is due to
the increase in fiber. Though it's a good thing to upgrade your fiber
intake, it is best to do it gradually. When this happens, I recommend that
you cut back on your fiber slightly and then gradually increase it again.
The good news is that the bloating and gas will pass as your body accli-
mates to the increase in fiber-rich food.

FATS AND CONDIMENTS

When you're making up a fat-burning meal, not all condiments are fat, but fat
is always considered a condiment. Think of all the fats you add to your food—
such as full-fat cheeses, butter, dressings, sauces, and the oil you cook with—as
flavorings only.

Fats

FAT	PORTION SIZE	
	Women	Men
All salad or cooking oils, including olive oil	1 tablespoon	1 tablespoon
Avocado/guacamole	2 ounces (¼ medium)	2½ ounces (½ medium)
Butter/ghee	1 tablespoon	1 tablespoon

FAT	PORTION SIZE	
	Women	Men
Cheese	½ ounce (1 slice)	½ ounce (1 slice)
Cream cheese	1 tablespoon	1 tablespoon
Mayonnaise	1 tablespoon	1 tablespoon
Nuts (almonds, walnuts, cashews)	1 ounce / ¼ cup (20–23 pieces)	1 ounce / ¼ cup (20–23 pieces)
Peanut or almond butter	1 tablespoon	1 tablespoon
Sour cream (carb-rich; low- or nonfat)	2 tablespoons	2 tablespoons
Sour cream (fat-rich; full fat)	1 tablespoon	1 tablespoon

Condiments (Spreads, Sauces, Syrups, and Gravies)

CONDIMENT	PORTION SIZE (Men and Women)
Barbecue sauce	2 tablespoons
Chutney	1 tablespoon
Cocktail sauce	¼ cup
Gravy	¼ cup
Peanut sauce	1 tablespoon
Pesto	1 tablespoon
Relish	2 tablespoons
Steak sauce	2 tablespoons
Sugar-free syrup	4 tablespoons / ¼ cup
Sweet-and-sour sauce	2 tablespoons
Sweet relish	2 tablespoons
Syrup (maple, rice)	1 tablespoon
Tahini	1 tablespoon
Tartar sauce	1 tablespoon
Tomato sauce	½ cup

Have as much as you want of any of the following condiments:

Fish sauce

Horseradish (without added
  sugar)

Hot pepper sauce (such as
  Tabasco)

Sugar-free jams and jellies

Lemon juice

Mustard

Pico de gallo

Salsa (excluding those made
  with beans or corn)

Sauerkraut

Low-sodium soy sauce

Tamari

Vinegar

Wasabi

Worcestershire (without added
  sugar)

▶ Alcohol and Fat Loss

WHEN YOU DRINK alcohol, your liver's priority function is the removal of the alcohol from your blood over all its other metabolic functions. The amounts of alcohol specified in the accompanying beverage chart are those the liver can process in 1 hour while still maintaining its other functions, one of which is metabolizing fat. So if you drink more than that, your liver will be devoting all its energies to dealing with the alcohol, which means that it will stop metabolizing fat. Therefore, when you drink too much, you are more likely to gain fat.

Beverages

BEVERAGE	PORTION SIZE (Men and Women)
Juices made from fast-carb fruits (orange juice)	8 ounces
Juices made from slow-carb fruits or vegetables (carrot juice)	12 ounces
Wine	5 ounces
Soda (sugared pop or soft drink) or beer	12 ounces
Soda (zero calorie)	unlimited
Liquor (scotch, bourbon, vodka, gin)	1½ ounces
Milk (all types, except coconut milk)	8 ounces

COFFE AND HOT and iced tea can be consumed in any quantity. (Watch the caffeine, however, if that is of concern to you.) When you add honey or half-and-half, they are classified as snacks, such as a skinny latte (140 calories).

When it comes to water, the key is to drink enough so that your urine is clear—and so that you never actually feel thirsty. The amount you drink to keep properly hydrated will depend on many factors including your body, level of activity, and climate.

How to Make a Fat-Burning Meal

There are three basic ways you can make a proper fat-burning meal. (Condiments and fat portions are not mentioned in the chart below but may be added as flavorings. Note that you need to be especially careful because all fats are calorically dense.)

1:1:1 RATIO	1 portion protein, 1 portion fast carbs, 1 portion slow carbs
	For example, turkey, baked potato, and a vegetable; *or* turkey, a vegetable, and a glass of wine; *or* spaghetti and meatballs and a side salad
	Because eating fast and slow carbs together slows down the rate at which you metabolize the fast carb, you get to eat one of each with your protein
1:3 RATIO	1 portion protein and 3 portions slow carbs
	For example, a big salad with grilled chicken on top, *or* a stir-fry of three vegetables and a portion of cube steak
	Because slow carbs are metabolized more slowly, you can eat two portions for every one portion of fast carbs
1:1 RATIO	1 portion protein and 1 portion fast carbs
	For example, scrambled eggs and toast, *or* steak and a baked potato
	Because fast carbs are metabolized quickly, you can eat only one portion when you're not also eating a slow carb to slow it down

Please note that you *must* have at least 15 grams of protein and 30 grams of carbs at every meal—and that includes breakfast. Otherwise you're eating a snack! We'll be talking all about snacks later in this chapter.

To make your fat-burning meal, all you have to do is decide which ratio you're going to have, what your protein is going to be, and what carb side you want to go with it. That's it—as easy as 1, 2, 3!

Fat Loss Fusion

A Fat Loss Fusion is a fat-burning meal in which proteins and carbs are combined in a single dish—such as chili, lasagna, a stew, or a casserole—the goal being to get your minimum of 15 grams of protein and not exceed the carb intake. The meals in the following chart provide several examples.

Dish	Ratio and Ingredients	Portion Size	
		Women	Men
Lasagna*	1:1:1	2 cups	2½ cups
	Protein: ground beef		
	Fast carb: pasta		
	Slow carb: vegetables or a side salad		
	Condiment: tomato sauce		
Beef stew	1:1:1	2 cups	2½ cups
	Protein: beef		
	Fast carb: potatoes		
	Slow carb: vegetables		
Chili	1:1:1	2 cups	2½ cups
	Protein: ground beef or turkey		
	Fast carb: side of elbow macaroni		
	Slow carb: beans		
	Condiment: tomato sauce		

*If you decide not to have the vegetables or side salad, this would be a 1:1 ratio meal.

THE SECRET OF SNACKING

To keep your blood sugar level and to maximize fat loss, you *must* snack. You're going to be eating at least two snacks (morning and afternoon) and perhaps even a third or fourth one if you eat dinner early and don't go to bed until late. Your snacks should come 2 to 3 hours after your previous meal and no later than 1 hour before you go to bed.

In addition to preventing your blood sugar levels from dropping too low, snacking helps you control hunger so that you're not tempted to binge at your next meal. In a study from Johannesburg, South Africa, published in the *International Journal of Obesity and Related Metabolic Disorders*, frequent meals reduced appetite by 27 percent and resulted in much more favorable insulin and blood glucose profiles.

Q Are there any foods or ingredients I should avoid or add to lose the most weight during the first 7 days and keep from gaining any unwanted pounds?—Mary O. (Kansas City, MO)

A Although I do emphasize that living diet-free does not involve deprivation, common sense dictates that certain products (sometimes called food) are obstructions to fat loss. The seven most common are the following:

- Products that have high fructose corn syrup listed in the first four ingredients
- Products that have enriched wheat flour listed in the first four ingredients
- Alcohol of all types
- Deep-fried foods of any kind
- Added salt to your food
- Frozen or prepared entrées that have more than 700 milligrams of sodium in a serving
- Products containing trans-fats and unhealthy fats, including partially hydrogenated oils, fractionated oils, lard, shortening, and interesterified fat

And another study by Scandinavian researchers published in the *European Journal of Clinical Nutrition* compared two groups of competitive boxers who were trying to lose weight by reducing their calorie intake. Both groups lost the same amount of weight, but those who ate two square meals a day lost more lean body mass than those who had six meals a day. Therefore: *It pays to snack!*

So how do you know what to snack on? That's easy: *pretty much anything you like.* A snack doesn't have to include a carb, but it can. In fact, you can snack on potato chips if that's what you like. And you don't have to worry about whether it's a fast carb or a slow carb because one portion isn't going to affect your blood sugar enough to throw you into fat-storing mode. There are only two guidelines for snacks.

- If it's a whole food—that is, if it's a piece of fruit, a chicken breast, a potato, or anything that doesn't come in a package, you can eat **one**

portion or as much as you need to consume **no fewer than 100 calories and no more than 200 calories (women) or 300 calories (men).** For example, 1 cup of carrots is not enough; you would have to eat at least 2 cups of carrots to get 100 calories.

- If it comes in a package and has a label, you can eat anything you want so long as it's between **100 and 200 calories for women** and **100 to 300 calories for men.**

That's it!

And I mean it. You can have your snack in the form of cookies so long as they are within the correct calorie range, and I actually recommend that you eat chocolate at least once a day.

▶ The Wine and Chocolate Snack

WE ALL KNOW that a nice glass of wine and a good piece of dark chocolate really make you feel good, and when you're living diet-free, you can have both.

A portion of chocolate is 1 ounce for women (about the size of two dominoes) and 1 to 2 ounces for men. Choose dark chocolate with at least 60 percent cocoa content when possible because it will have the least amount of sugar. When the packaging doesn't indicate the cocoa content, choose the one that is highest in fat compared to sugar or carbs.

A portion of good dark chocolate and a 5-ounce glass of red or white wine makes a great 180- to 200-calorie snack. On average, both red and white wine yield about 20 calories per ounce.

Now you have all the basics, but you'll want to make sure your newfound fat loss method works for you. That's what you're going to be doing in the following chapter.

7

Customize Your Plan So That It Works for You

To truly live diet-free, you have to take charge. And even though I can be your coach, it's time for you to move into the driver's seat.

CREATE YOUR PERSONAL MEAL PLAN

Now is the time to start putting all your preparation into action. So get out your journal and start to write up a menu that works for you.

I've had clients from Puerto Rico to Egypt to Alaska to Austria, all of whom have easily adapted diet-free living to their own preferences. So the first thing for you to do is to make a list of all the foods that you eat most often and that you enjoy. Check your list against my lists of proteins, fast carbs, slow carbs, fats, and condiments to determine into which category they fall. Once you've done that, you'll be able to start making fat-burning meals to suit your personal palate. To start you off, I suggest that you come up with menus for 7 days of breakfasts, lunches, and dinners.

As examples, here are ideas for three breakfasts, lunches, and dinners. Feel free to use them, adjust them, or ignore them and create your own.

Breakfast 1

Egg white omelet (protein) with mushrooms, tomatoes, and peppers (slow carb)

Two slices of whole wheat toast (fast carb) topped with 1 tablespoon butter (fat) and jam (condiment)

Breakfast 2

Smoothie made with 1 scoop vanilla protein powder (protein) blended with ½ banana (½ portion fast carb), 4 ounces milk (½ portion fast carb), 1 cup berries (slow carb), 1 tablespoon natural peanut butter (fat), and enough water to reach your desired consistency.

Breakfast 3

Cereal (fast carb) with 1 cup milk (fast carb). When you combine a serving of cereal (serving size based on the recommendation on the package) with 1 cup milk, you are creating a Fat Loss Fusion. I recommend that you choose a cereal with at least 4 grams of protein and 4 grams of fiber. If your cereal has 4 grams of protein and you combine it with milk, your total yield is 11 grams of protein. And as long as you don't exceed the recommended number of carbs, you have created a fat-burning meal.

Lunch 1

Hamburger (protein) with lettuce (all-you-want raw vegetables), tomato (slow carb), and mustard (condiment) on a bun (fast carb)

Lunch 2

Grilled fish (protein), black beans (slow carb), and fries (fast carb)

Lunch 3

Chicken salad (protein) with mixed vegetables (slow carb)

Dinner 1

Grilled chicken (protein) with pinto beans (slow carb), carrots (slow carb), and a side salad (all-you-want raw vegetables)

Dinner 2

Sliced turkey (protein) with mashed potatoes (fast carb), asparagus (slow carb), and a large salad (all-you-want raw vegetables)

Dinner 3

Steak (protein), 1 glass wine (fast carb), a large salad (all-you-want raw vegetables), and broccoli (slow carb)

If you're not feeling creative or would like other suggestions, see the recipes in Chapter 11, which were created to enhance your fat loss dining experience.

Record your planned meals in your journal, and remember to leave enough space between each meal to enter your snacks.

You can always make changes later on if you have to. Maybe you decided early in the week that you were going to have meatballs and spaghetti on Friday, but then you went to an Italian restaurant on Tuesday and had your meatballs and spaghetti meal then. That's okay. You can move the meal you'd planned to eat on Tuesday to Friday, or you can choose an entirely different meal for that day.

Remember, this is *your* menu plan; you created it in the first place, so you're allowed to change it—so long as your changes stay within the guidelines for making a fat-burning meal.

CUSTOMIZED SNACKING

A snack can be anything you want to eat, from an apple to a bag of chips, so long as it contains between 100 and 200 calories for women and 100 to 300 calories for men. If you're in any doubt about how many calories your snack might have, check one of the Internet calorie counters (for example, www .nutritiondata.com or www.calorieking.com). Or purchase a pocket-size guide at any bookstore.

Don't skip your snacks! Eating something every 2 to 3 hours is as important to your fat loss success as eating the proper combination of protein, fast carbs, and slow carbs at every meal. So plan your snacks as well as your meals and write them in your journal.

FAQ

Q Can I eat a banana with my cereal in the morning, or do I need to wait the 2 to 3 hours after the cereal and make it a snack? —Margaret K. (Keene, NH)

A When eating breakfast, you don't want to consume two fast carbs together (with the exception of milk and cereal). I recommend that if you want fruit in your cereal, add some berries, which are slow carbs, and eat the banana for a snack.

Here are just a few of the virtually unlimited kinds of snacks you could choose from:

- One portion of any whole fruit (see lists in Chapter 6)
- One portion of any whole protein (see lists in Chapter 6)
- A slice of toast with 1 tablespoon peanut butter or cream cheese
- Chips or pretzels
- One portion of nuts (20 to 23)
- Yogurt
- A small can of Albacore tuna
- An ice cream bar or sandwich

As long as it's in your calorie range and feels okay for your body, it's an okay snack.

Now, record your planned snacks in your journal.

I'M NOT ABOUT to renege on my promise that if you haven't been exercising, you don't have to start the first week. But if you are doing some kind of exercise already, you need to know how to combine eating and exercise in a way that will maximize your fat loss and help you increase your lean body tissue.

■ ALL EXERCISE

1. Except for first thing in the morning, you should eat a meal or a snack 30 to 40 minutes before your workout. Make it a habit to wait at least 30 minutes after eating so that you can digest your food before you exercise.

2. Your preexercise snack should have more carbs than protein but should contain at least 5 to 10 grams of protein whenever possible.

3. Always eat a meal or a snack within 1 hour after completing your workout.

■ LIGHT CARDIO EXERCISE: WALKING, SWIMMING, BIKING, AEROBICS CLASS

1. If you are going to do light cardio exercise within 60 minutes of when you get up, you don't need to eat first—unless you have a particular medical condition, such as diabetes, glucose intolerance, or hypoglycemia. Drinking coffee, tea, or water before exercising on an empty stomach is perfectly okay. In fact, studies have shown that caffeine can boost your metabolism and contribute to exercise performance.

2. If you exercise on an empty stomach, be sure to eat breakfast within 1 hour after completing your workout. Then continue eating every 2 to 3 hours until 1 hour before bedtime.

(continued)

■ RESISTANCE TRAINING

1. If you are going to lift weights within an hour of getting up, eat a pre-workout snack that contains carbohydrates in addition to at least 5 to 10 grams of protein, such as a slice of toast with 1 tablespoon peanut butter and jam with no sugar added.

2. Eat breakfast within 1 hour of completing your workout, and then eat something every 2 to 3 hours until 1 hour before bedtime.

MAKE A LIST AND GO SHOPPING

Once you have your food plan in place, make a shopping list for the week and be sure you've got everything you're going to need in the pantry or the refrigerator. Just as you don't want to get up and brush your teeth while trying to figure out what you'll be having for breakfast, you don't want to go into the kitchen and discover that you've run out of your favorite cereal or that the eggs you thought you had aren't there anymore.

Planning in advance is one way to eliminate one source of stress—and also one excuse we might have for not following the plan.

Realtor and mother of four Kim L. has a crazy schedule. Initially, when she explained her stressful lifestyle, she asked me, "What one thing—if there is a one thing—is going to help me achieve success in losing this weight?" My answer: "If you fail to plan, you plan to fail." Kim took my advice to heart, and in the first 8 weeks she lost 30 pounds. She stuck with the plan and the planning and went on to lose more than 80 pounds altogether, and her teenage son, Ethan, lost 100 pounds.

WHEN LIFE GETS IN THE WAY

Even the best-laid plans can fall by the wayside when the unexpected occurs. Maybe your alarm failed to go off (or you forgot to set it) and you don't have time for a meal before you leave for work. Maybe you have lunch out one day instead of eating at home or at your desk. Or maybe you're invited out to dinner.

Any plan that's going to work has to be flexible enough to adapt to change.

Adapting Your Snack When You Can't Eat a Meal

If you're forced to skip a meal, you'll need to rethink your snacking to prevent your metabolism from slowing and your blood sugar from dropping so low that you start to store rather than burn fat. What this means is that a pure protein snack might not do the trick. Instead, you may need to eat a combination of protein and carbs both to keep yourself feeling full and to keep your blood sugar level from dropping.

In the end, each one of us is unique, and no two bodies process nutrients exactly the same way, so you need to pay attention to how you feel. As you follow the menu plan, you'll become more aware of your personal energy needs.

Take Bella, for instance. She was eating high-protein snacks with little or no carbs because she'd decided that she didn't want to lose any lean muscle tissue, and since she was eating carbs at meals, she thought that snacking on protein would be the right way to go. The problem was that she felt tired and lacking in energy every afternoon. At first she thought she was hypoglycemic (had low blood sugar) and that there wasn't much she could do about it. But when I looked at her food journal, I realized that she was desperately lacking in carbs. By replacing her afternoon snack with a piece of fruit or an energy bar that was higher in carbs than protein, she magically stopped experiencing those afternoon energy drops and continued to progress with her fat loss.

Some of us can have protein-rich snacks without experiencing major drops in blood sugar, while others need carb-rich snacks to keep blood sugar levels from dropping too low. Over time, you will discover what works best for your own body and energy needs.

Eating Out

Eating in a restaurant is challenging for almost anyone who's trying to lose weight, but being able to live diet-free means learning how to adapt your choices to just about any dining experience.

General Guidelines

- Keep in mind that restaurant portions are almost always larger than those recommended for the fat-burning meal. When your food arrives, eyeball your portion and ask your server to bring a doggie bag *before* you begin eating. That way the extra food will be out of sight and you'll have a second fat-burning meal to eat the next day.
- Grilled meat or poultry or grilled or steamed fish is almost always a good protein choice. Just remember to ask for the sauce on the side.
- A baked potato, pasta with a tomato-based sauce, or rice are all generally available fast carb choices.
- Your slow carb could be grilled or steamed vegetables, beans, or a salad with the dressing on the side.

▶ The Psychology of Eating Out

IF YOU DIDN'T already know this, let me tell you that you're greedy. Yes, that's what I said. I'm greedy, and practically all of us are greedy when it comes to most things in life—especially food. So, let me ask you this question: If I offered you either a loaf of bread or a single slice for $1, which would you choose? No-brainer, right? If you could get more for your money, you'd take it. Well, that's also true when it comes to eating out. Even if you don't ultimately get drawn in by the fact that you can get two burgers for $1 or that you save money when you accept the supersize offer, you are bound to be tempted because it's nice to save money.

Therefore, when you're eating out, it is important that you know what you want before you order and then stick to your guns. I know deals are nice, but they can also prove disastrous to your waistline. Even if you're offered a complimentary add-on, unless you can bag it for a snack later or give it to someone else, just say no thank you, and you'll be happy you didn't get sucked in psychologically.

Italian Restaurant Choices

- Proteins: grilled meat, fish, shrimp, or chicken
- Fast carbs: pasta, risotto, potato, wine

- Slow carbs: steamed, sautéed, or grilled vegetables; salad with dressing on the side
- Fat Loss Fusion: lasagna or pizza

Chinese Restaurant Choices
- Proteins: steamed or stir-fried chicken or shrimp with vegetables (sauce on the side); shrimp or lobster Cantonese
- Fast carbs: steamed white or brown rice; steamed dumplings
- Slow carbs: steamed or stir-fried vegetables
- Fat Loss Fusion: moo goo gai pan (stir-fried white-meat chicken with mushrooms and other slow-carb vegetables, served with a light sauce made from chicken broth)
- Ask for your dishes to be prepared without added sugar, salt, or MSG; go easy on condiments such as hoisin sauce, and ask for low-sodium soy sauce.

Japanese Restaurant Choices
- Proteins: sashimi; steamed or grilled meat, poultry, or fish; tofu
- Fast carbs: steamed rice; udon or soba noodles
- Slow carbs: steamed, sautéed, or grilled vegetables
- Fat Loss Fusion: chicken sukiyaki (with the dipping sauce on the side)
- Ask for low-sodium soy sauce.

Mexican Restaurant Choices
- Proteins: chicken, steak, or shrimp fajitas; grilled or broiled fish, chicken, or lean red meat
- Fast carbs: rice, corn, tortillas
- Slow carbs: green salad; steamed, sautéed, or grilled vegetables; beans; vegetarian refried beans
- Fat Loss Fusion: chicken quesadilla (ask your waiter to go light on the cheese)
- Ask for such extras as cheese and sour cream to be served on the side. Use salsa instead of guacamole as a condiment; avoid the fried chips that are almost always put on the table before you even order your meal.
- If you're having an alcoholic beverage as your fast carb, stick with beer or wine and avoid the high-calorie, salty margarita.

Fast-Food Restaurant Choices

- Regular (not supersize) grilled chicken, fish, or roast beef sandwich with lettuce and tomato (dressing on the side)
- Regular (not supersize) hamburger on a bun with lettuce and tomato and 2 tablespoons ketchup
- Green salad with dressing on the side (or use lemon juice instead)

▶ Why You Need to Eat Your Bun

ONE OF MY actress/comedian clients called to tell me that I'd be very proud of her because she had gone to McDonald's, ordered a fish sandwich, and eaten only half the bun.

Unfortunately, I had to give her the not-so-positive news that she'd have been better off eating the whole bun because she hadn't had enough carbs to make a proper fat-burning meal, which meant that she had actually put herself at risk of lowering her blood sugar level and going into fat-storage mode.

Again, eating *enough* of *all* your macronutrients is just as important as not eating too much. Without the proper balance of protein, fast carbs, and slow carbs, you're eating a snack, not a meal. Although, as I have said, you may have to substitute a snack for a meal once in a while, meals and snacks are not intended to be interchangeable.

DON'T WANT TO THINK ABOUT IT?

Although the majority of my clients embrace the idea that they can choose the foods they want to eat, some just want me to give them a diet to follow so that they don't have to think about it. If you're one of those people who don't have the time or simply don't want to have to plan your meals and snacks, don't worry; what follows are sample menu plans with seven options each for breakfast, lunch, dinner, and snacks for both men and women.

Fresh Start for Men

These Fresh Start eating suggestions helped 26-year-old Kevin, who is single, constantly working, and always eating out, lose 9 pounds in 7 days, going from 265 to 256.

Breakfast

1. Kashi Go Lean Crunch cereal (1 serving) with 8 ounces milk.*
2. Kashi Heart to Heart Cereal (1 serving) with EAS AdvantEdge Carb Control french vanilla shake.
3. Smoothie made with protein powder (15 to 25 grams per serving), ½ banana, 4 ounces milk, 1 tablespoon natural peanut butter, and 1 cup blueberries.
4. Egg white or egg substitute (5 to 6 egg whites) omelet with tomatoes, bell peppers, mushrooms, spinach, and light cheese (no more than 1 ounce); two slices sourdough bread topped with 1 tablespoon nut butter (peanut butter, almond butter) and jam (no more than 2 tablespoons).
5. Protein-rich, nonfat Greek yogurt (1 cup) mixed with 1 banana and 1 cup berries (strawberries, blueberries).
6. Carb-rich yogurt (1 cup) eaten with a protein-rich energy bar.
7. Oatmeal (1 cup cooked) mixed with 15 to 25 grams protein powder and 1 cup of sliced strawberries.

Q I have switched from skim milk to unsweetened almond milk (I don't like soy milk), but almond milk doesn't have much protein in it. Should I add another protein source to my breakfast meal? —Andrea C. (Chico, CA)

A You could choose a breakfast cereal that is high in protein to make up for the reduced amount in a cup of almond milk. You could also substitute an EAS AdvantEdge Carb Control shake, which has 17 grams of protein in a single serving, for the almond milk. I would also recommend adding 2 or 3 egg whites or 1 whole egg and maybe even a meatless patty to your meal to get that minimum of 15 grams of protein when you use almond milk.

FAQ

*Any milk except coconut milk.

Morning (or Afternoon) Snack

1. Clif ZBar.

2. Clif energy bar.

3. Piece of fruit (pear, apple, banana).

4. Nuts (20–23; almonds, cashews).

5. Albacore tuna (2 small cans).

6. Chicken breast (5 to 6 ounces).

7. Turkey slices (5 to 6 ounces).

Lunch

1. Burrito made with egg whites (5 to 6 whites) and slow-carb mixed vegetables (tomatoes, spinach) wrapped in a tortilla.

2. Sandwich made with chicken, turkey, or a Boca burger patty (6 ounces); 2 slices bread; lettuce; tomatoes; light cheese (1 slice or no more than 1 ounce); and a mustard spread.

3. Grilled chicken (6 ounces) with 1 baked potato.

4. Sushi roll with yellowtail, Albacore tuna, or salmon (6 ounces), and a side salad.

5. Turkey (6 ounces) sandwich on honey oat bread from Subway, packed with slow carbs (peppers) and a mustard spread.

6. Steak (4 ounces) with rice (½ to ⅔ cup) and beans (½ to ⅔ cup).

7. Two fish tacos with beans (½ to ⅔ cup) and side salad.

Dinner

1. Chicken salad at Mexican restaurant with balsamic vinaigrette dressing.

2. Chicken (6 ounces) wrapped in lettuce leaf with a side salad of slow-carb vegetables.

3. Turkey salad with balsamic vinaigrette dressing.

4. Chicken (6 ounces) and slow-carb veggie stir-fry (3 cups of vegetables).

5. Egg white frittata with mixed slow-carb vegetables (broccoli, spinach, mushrooms, peppers).

6. Grilled fish (6 ounces; tilapia, halibut, trout) with asparagus (7 to 8 stalks or a hand-size portion).

7. Protein-rich smoothie made with EAS AdvantEdge Carb Control french vanilla shake, 1 tablespoon peanut butter, 1 scoop protein powder, and 2 cups berries (blueberries, strawberries).

Evening Snack

1. EAS AdvantEdge Carb Control shake (any flavor).
2. Nuts (20–23; almonds, cashews).
3. Albacore tuna (2 small cans).
4. Chicken breast (5 to 6 ounces).
5. Turkey slices (5 to 6 ounces).
6. Cottage cheese (1 cup) with 1 cup berries (blueberries, strawberries).
7. Protein-rich smoothie made with protein powder, ½ cup berries (blueberries, strawberries), and EAS AdvantEdge Carb Control shake (any flavor).

Fresh Start for Women

Lynn, a 47-year-old wife and mother of three children, lost 5 pounds in the first 7 days, going from 173 to 168, following these eating suggestions.

Breakfast

1. Kashi Heart to Heart cereal (1 serving) with 8 ounces milk.*
2. Kashi Heart to Heart cereal (1 serving) with EAS AdvantEdge Carb Control french vanilla shake.
3. Smoothie made with protein powder (15 to 25 grams per serving), ½ banana, 4 ounces milk, 1 tablespoon natural peanut butter, and 1 cup blueberries.
4. Whole egg with 2 egg whites scrambled, and 2 slices sourdough bread topped with 1 tablespoon peanut butter and 2 tablespoons jam.
5. Protein-rich, nonfat Greek yogurt (1 cup) mixed with 2 cups berries (strawberries, blueberries).
6. Starbucks strawberry/banana Vivanno smoothie made with soy milk.
7. Oatmeal (1 cup cooked) mixed with 15 to 25 grams protein powder, sweetened with sugar-free syrup and topped with 23 walnuts.

_____

*Any milk except coconut milk.

Morning Snack

1. Energy bar (Clif ZBar or Mojo, Luna).
2. Piece of fruit (pear, apple, banana).
3. Nuts (20–23; almonds, cashews).
4. EAS AdvantEdge Carb Control shake (any flavor).
5. Protein-rich, nonfat Greek yogurt (1 cup) sweetened with 1 tablespoon vanilla protein powder.
6. Microwave popcorn (100 calories).
7. V8 juice (12 ounces).

Lunch

1. Fish (4 ounces; tilapia, halibut, trout, salmon) with sautéed slow-carb vegetables (3 cups).
2. Steak (3 ounces) with potato (fist size) or ½ cup brown rice, and 1 cup broccoli.
3. Turkey (4 ounces) sandwich with lettuce, tomato, and mustard spread on whole wheat bread.
4. Chicken breast (5 ounces), ½ cup steamed corn or brown rice, and ½ cup pinto beans.
5. Chicken breast (5 ounces) with 3 cups slow-carb steamed vegetables.
6. Grilled mahi mahi (5 ounces) on a plate full of salad.
7. Pan-fried tilapia (5 ounces) with ½ cup brown rice and ½ cup black beans.

Afternoon Snack

1. Energy bar (Clif's ZBar or Mojo, Luna).
2. Piece of fruit (pear, apple, banana).
3. Nuts (20–23; almonds, cashews).
4. Rice cakes (2 cakes), each topped with ½ tablespoon natural peanut butter.
5. Protein-rich, nonfat Greek yogurt (1 cup) sweetened with 1 tablespoon vanilla protein powder.
6. Microwave popcorn (100 calories).
7. Whole grapefruit.

Dinner

1. Shrimp (5 ounces) and salad with 2 cups slow-carb vegetables mixed in.
2. Chicken breast (5 ounces) sliced over plate full of salad with glycemic easy Fat-Burning Salad Dressing (recipe on page 213).
3. Albacore tuna (2 small cans; 8 ounces total) on a bed of sliced tomatoes.
4. Albacore tuna (1 small can) over medium baked/mashed yam with mustard spread.
5. Burrito made with whole wheat tortilla, chicken breast (5 ounces), ½ cup black beans, sliced tomato, ½ ounce reduced-fat cheese, and hot sauce.
6. Egg whites (5) scrambled with 2 cups slow-carb vegetables and served over a bed of lettuce.
7. Corn tortillas (2) with chicken breast (5 ounces), ¼ cup black beans, ¼ cup tomatoes, and ½ ounce shredded cheese, topped with ½ cup nonfat Greek yogurt.

Evening Snack

1. Energy bar (Clif's ZBar or Mojo, Luna).
2. EAS AdvantEdge Carb Control shake (any flavor).
3. Nuts (20–23; almonds, cashews).
4. Rice cakes (2 cakes), each topped with ½ tablespoon natural peanut butter.
5. Protein-rich, nonfat Greek yogurt (1 cup) sweetened with 1 tablespoon vanilla protein powder.
6. Microwave popcorn (100 calories).
7. Whole grapefruit.

8

Fat Loss for Vegetarians

Many people believe that if they simply stop eating meat they will automatically lose weight. Not true! I was a vegan for almost 12 years while also being a professional mixed martial artist. Because I was so active and was training on an elite level, I remained lean and healthy, but most people I know who are vegan or vegetarian and not so active are overweight, have a hard time losing weight, or look a bit gaunt because they're not getting enough protein and are therefore lacking in lean muscle tissue.

My own mother decided at one point to become a vegetarian because she thought that cutting out animal products would put her on the path to weight loss; instead, she gained 50 pounds in less than 6 months.

Stephani R., a vegetarian, wasn't overweight by most people's standards, but as an avid runner and fitness enthusiast, she couldn't figure out why, considering her active lifestyle, she wasn't able to lose weight. Stephani attended one of my favorite seminars, which I call "The Fat Vegetarian," and after learning how to combine her foods so that she was getting adequate amounts of protein and not too many carbs, she dropped 30 pounds, going from 145 pounds to a fit 115, and her body fat went from 33 to 18 percent. In her words: "I've been a vegetarian for more than twenty years and spent thousands on weight loss courses and personal trainers and then I met Robert Ferguson. His simple recommendations helped me drop thirty pounds quickly. I still enjoy all of my favorite foods but thanks to Robert, I now have the tools I need to stay lean and healthy for the rest of my life."

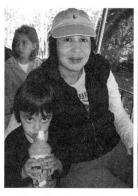 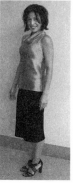

Stephani R. dropped 7 pounds in the first 7 days and averaged a little more than 2 pounds a week until she reached her goal weight of 115.

▶ Famous Vegetarian Athletes

Billie Jean King, tennis player

Carl Lewis, track and field

Edwin Moses, track and field

Joe Namath, quarterback for the New York Jets

Martina Navratilova, tennis player

Robert Parish, center for the Boston Celtics

Bill Pearl, Mr. Universe

Dave Scott, six-time winner of the Iron Man Triathlon

WHY VEGETARIANS GET FAT

The problem for many vegetarians is that because they've cut out the most obvious and available sources of protein—specifically meat, poultry, and fish—their diet consists mainly of carbs and fat. And, as you now know, flooding your system with too many carbs triggers the production of insulin and throws your body into fat-storing mode. The key is to learn how to get enough protein on a daily basis without consuming too many carbs.

Some people who don't eat meat or poultry do eat fish, which is, of course, a really good protein source. Others—the majority—are ovo-lacto vegetarians, meaning that they eat eggs and dairy products. They, too, have a relatively easy time with protein but may wind up eating too much fat. Eggs, milk, and cheese are all sources of complete protein, meaning that they provide all the essential amino acids your body can't manufacture for itself, but they can also be high in fat. So eating primarily egg whites, skim milk, or reduced-fat cheese is a good way to get your protein without too much fat.

The strictest vegetarians—that is, vegans—don't eat any foods that come from animals or contain animal-source products, and that includes eggs and dairy products. Since the only vegetable sources of complete protein are soy and quinoa, vegans have the hardest time getting all the protein they need without overdoing their intake of carbs. But with the right information, that problem, too, can be solved.

When I met Kelley, she weighed 258 pounds and was at the point where she believed the only way she could lose weight was to undergo Lap-Band surgery. Because she was a vegan and ate only organic foods that were close to nature, Kelley believed she was following a healthy diet and couldn't understand why she wasn't able to lose weight.

After looking at what she ate on a daily basis and calculating her calorie and carbohydrate intake for a day, I understood only too well where her problem lay. For example, one of Kelley's lunch favorites was a bowl of pasta with marinara sauce, French bread with rice cheese and hummus, a large salad, and sweetened tea. This meal alone had more than 100 grams of carbohydrates and fewer than 10 grams of protein. And because she went for long periods of time without eating, sometimes that meal wasn't enough to satisfy her and she'd have a little more pasta.

We replaced the French bread with a whole wheat roll to give her a couple of additional grams of protein, kept her pasta portion to 2 cups and the marinara to ¼ cup, and left her tea unsweetened. I also suggested that she keep a packet of protein powder in her purse so that she could mix it with water and drink it to get an additional 12 grams of protein. To help her feel full, she doubled the amount of hummus she put on her roll. Without having to change her habits drastically, Kelley was able to get more than 20 grams of protein into her favorite meal while also lowering her carbs-minus-fiber total to 40 to 45 grams. In addition, she made sure to have a snack 2 hours before eating her favorite lunch and another 3 hours after.

Kelley, who had been considering surgery, went from 258 pounds to 144 pounds in just over a year. She is still a vegan and now understands how to combine carbohydrates and fat in a way that provides her with the protein she needs. And because she's chosen the vegan lifestyle, she's willing to support that choice by looking up the caloric and nutrient content of various foods when she needs to in order to be sure she's making a proper fat loss plate.

▶ Worried About Complete Protein?

PEOPLE WHO EAT eggs and dairy, as I've said, don't really have to worry.

- 1 large egg white contains 3.6 grams of complete protein and 0.2 gram of carbs.
- 1 ounce of Kraft Cheddar cheese contains 7 grams of complete protein and 1 gram of carbs.
- 1 cup (8 ounces) of skim milk contains 8.7 grams of complete protein and 12.3 grams of carbs.

THOSE WHO GET all their protein strictly from plant sources (other than soy and quinoa) need to eat a variety of foods to get all the essential amino acids found in complete proteins. But even that isn't very difficult.

You don't need to get all the essential amino acids at every meal. In fact, according to Madelyn Fernstrom, director of the Weight Management Center at the Pittsburgh Medical Center, "Children should try to get as complete an assortment of amino acids as they can on a weekly basis. Adults should aim to get all their amino acids on a monthly basis. We *do* have a biological drive to seek protein to satisfy our bodies' needs, so there is little likelihood we will have deficiencies. But balance is key."

It is interesting that the combinations of foods that make up complete proteins are those we tend to eat together anyway: peanut butter on whole wheat bread; rice and beans; hummus (chickpeas and sesame paste).

The bottom line is that if you're getting a sufficient amount of protein at each meal and you're eating a variety of foods (fruits, whole grains, vegetables) throughout the day, you really don't have to worry very much about whether the protein is complete or not.

How to Make a Vegetarian Fat-Burning Meal

When you're making a vegetarian fat-burning meal, the guidelines for specific nutrients still apply. You need to have:

- *At least* 15 grams of protein
- *No more than* 45 grams of carbohydrates for women and 50 grams for men after you subtract the total fiber

As I mentioned earlier, unless you eat fish, eggs, or soy products, you will be obtaining your protein from carb sources, so you'll need to be aware of how many grams of protein and how many grams of carbs there are in the foods you choose. Once you know that, you can easily combine them to make a fat-burning meal. The following chart lists some common protein-rich vegetarian foods along with their protein and carb content.

Protein-Rich Vegetarian Foods

FOOD	VEGETARIAN SERVING SIZE	PROTEIN (GRAMS)	CARBS (GRAMS)*	FIBER (GRAMS)
Almonds, whole kernels	1 ounce, 23 nuts	6.0	6.0	3.5
Beans, black	½ cup cooked	7.5	13.0	7.5
Beans, kidney	½ cup cooked	7.6	20.1	5.7
Beans, refried	½ cup cooked	6.4	16.3	5.7
Broccoli	1 cup chopped, cooked	3.7	11.2	5.1
Chickpeas	½ cup cooked	7.5	22.5	6.2
Kale	1 cup cooked	3.7	6.8	2.6
Lentils, mature seeds	½ cup cooked	8.9	19.9	7.8
Oatmeal, instant (Quaker Oats)	1 cup cooked	5.9	25.5	4.0
Pasta (Barilla)	1 cup cooked	6.7	35.5	2.1
Peanut butter (natural)	2 tablespoons	8.0	7.6	2.0
Potato, red	1 medium, baked	4.0	33.9	3.1
Potato, white	1 medium, baked	4.3	36.7	3.8
Quinoa	½ cup cooked	4.0	19.5	2.5
Rice, long-grain, brown	½ cup cooked	2.5	22.3	1.8
Rice, long-grain, white	½ cup cooked	2.0	22.3	0.3
Soybeans, green, raw	½ cup cooked	16.6	14.1	5.4
Soymilk, plain (Silk)	1 cup	7.0	8.0	1.0

*All carb grams are calculated after deducting the fiber content.

FOOD	VEGETARIAN SERVING SIZE	PROTEIN (GRAMS)	CARBS (GRAMS)*	FIBER (GRAMS)
Spinach	1 cup cooked	5.3	6.8	4.3
Sunflower seeds, hulled	¼ cup	6.9	7.7	3.6
Sweet potato	1 medium, baked	3.6	37.3	5.9
Tempeh	3 ounces cooked	15.5	8.0	0.0
Tofu, silken, extra firm	1 slice	6.0	1.7	0.1
Veggie hot dog	1 link	6.5	4.9	0.8
Walnuts	½ ounce, 7 halves	2.2	1.0	1.0
Yam	1 medium, baked	2.6	47	6.7

In some cases, the portion sizes given in the chart are larger than those on the food lists in Chapter 6. And in some cases, you may find that you're increasing the designated portion size (such as eating ¾ cup black beans instead of ½ cup). That's because you may need to eat more of a vegetable-based food to obtain adequate protein, and that's okay, so long as you don't exceed the total number of carb grams recommended in any given meal.

EDUCATE YOURSELF

Because the world we live in isn't really set up to accommodate vegetarians, becoming a diet-free vegetarian takes a bit of self-education. You can't, for example, go into a restaurant and order just a fruit plate, because you'd be getting way too many carbs and not enough protein. For example:

> 1 medium banana = 23.8 grams carbs (after deducting fiber) and 1.3 grams protein.
> 1 medium orange = 12.8 grams carbs (after deducting fiber) and 1.0 grams protein.
> 1 medium apple = 20.7 grams carbs (after deducting fiber) and 0.5 grams protein.

So, a fruit plate made up of 1 banana, 1 orange, and 1 apple would contain 57.3 grams of carbs, which is 12.3 more than recommended for women, and 7.3 more than what is recommended for men.

Now, look at the list of high-protein vegetarian foods in the preceding chart, and see how they can be combined with one another as well as with other foods to make a fat-burning plate. Note that all carb grams are calculated after deducting for fiber. The following examples will give a real sense of what I mean.

EXAMPLE 1: Peanut Butter and Jelly Sandwich on Whole Wheat Bread

2 tablespoons peanut butter = 8 grams protein and 5.6 grams carbs

2 slices whole wheat bread = 10 grams protein and 32 grams carbs

Jelly = condiment

Total: 18 grams protein and 37.6 grams carbs

EXAMPLE 2: Spinach Salad with Chanterelle Mushrooms, Walnuts, and Feta Cheese and Two Slices Whole Wheat Bread

2 cups raw spinach = 1.7 grams protein and 2.2 grams carbs

1 cup mushrooms = 2.2 grams protein and 1.6 grams carbs

½ ounce walnuts = 2.2 grams protein and 1 gram carbs

½ cup crumbled Feta cheese = 10.7 grams protein and 3 grams carbs

2 slices whole wheat bread = 10 grams protein and 32 grams carbs

Total: 26.8 grams protein[*] and 39.8 grams carbs

EXAMPLE 3: Whole Wheat Burrito with Black Beans, Salsa, and Avocado

1 large low-carb tortilla = 8 grams protein and 19 grams carbs

¾ cup black beans = 11.25 grams protein and 19.5 grams carbs

½ cup cubed avocado = 1.5 grams protein and 6.2 grams carbs

¼ cup salsa = 1 gram protein and 4 grams carbs

Total: 21.75 grams protein and 48.7 grams carbs

EXAMPLE 4: Quinoa with Portobello Mushrooms Sautéed in Olive Oil

1 cup cooked quinoa = 8 grams protein and 34 grams carbs

2 cups grilled portobello mushroom = 8 grams protein and 10.7 grams carbs

---

[*]Your body can process only so much protein at a time, about 30 grams for women and 40 grams for men. It's okay to exceed your protein intake when you're losing weight so long as it doesn't exceed 30 percent of your daily food intake.

1 tablespoons extra virgin olive oil = 0 grams protein and 0 grams carbs

Total: 16 grams protein and 44.7 grams carbs

EXAMPLE 5: Falafel in Whole Wheat Pita Bread Topped with Tahini

6 (2-inch) falafel patties = 13.5 grams protein and 32.5 grams carbs

1 small whole wheat pita = 3 grams protein and 15 grams carbs

1 tablespoon tahini = 3 grams protein and 4 grams carbs

Total: 19.5 grams protein and 52.5 grams carbs

There are many good books and many websites that will give you the nutritional content of most common (and not so common) foods. As I mentioned earlier, the websites I use most often are www.calorieking.com and www.nutritiondata.com. You can also download the USDA's database for nutritional data. After a while, you'll become more familiar with your favorite combinations and will find that you're no longer looking things up as often as you were when you started the plan.

FAT LOSS VEGETARIAN RECIPES

I have included a range of vegetarian recipes in Chapter 11, which have been marked with a special icon (V). Each recipe includes a complete nutritional breakdown of protein, carbohydrates, fiber, and fat, as well as a note about why I've chosen these combinations.

9

The 21-Day Mindset Makeover

Because living diet-free is as much a state of mind as it is a way of life, I'll be giving you a specific concept to focus on for each of the 21 days you've committed to changing the way you think about nutrition and fitness.

As each new thought builds on the ones that preceded it, your mind will gradually be opened to a whole new way of looking at yourself and how you choose to approach nutrition and health.

Before you begin, however, I want to let you know that I don't expect you to follow the makeover perfectly any more than I expect you to achieve total perfection in any other aspect of your life. What I'm giving you here is a road map, but as we all know, when you're on a journey, it's sometimes necessary to take a detour or make a rest stop. That's perfectly okay. Just do the best you can to stay on course and you'll get there in the end—at your own speed and in your own time.

DAY 1 ▶
DECIDE TO SUCCEED

> To see a thing clearly in the mind makes it begin to take form.
> —HENRY FORD

If there is a secret weapon that leads to the achievement of anything worthwhile, it is the mind. Behavioral specialists agree that whatever is impressed in your mind is expressed in reality. Therefore, if you *decide* to succeed, it will be only a matter of time before you achieve your desired weight loss.

I want you to decide *today*. People put off making decisions because they fear the unknown or that they will fail. Don't procrastinate; don't put it off for another minute. Announce out loud to yourself that you have made up your mind to live diet-free. There is no downside when you make that decision, even if you don't yet know *how* you're going to do it.

To make a conscious decision about something is to set your mind on the achievement of a specific outcome. As you continue to nurture your mindset for the next 21 days, you will be ensuring that the intentions you made manifest in your body.

Now take a few minutes to write down in your journal three decisions you have made that will support your intention to lose weight and keep it off. These may include trying one or more of the recipes in this book, finding 10 minutes a day to read something positive that will reinforce your new mindset, or simply continuing to follow the concepts in this book.

Once you've made the big decision—to succeed at living diet-free for life—every other decision you make becomes a guide post, a short-term goal, or a course correction that will help you stay on track.

▶ Fresh Start Reminder

DID YOU REMEMBER to eat breakfast within 30 to 60 minutes of getting up this morning?

Revving up your metabolism with a fat-burning meal in the morning puts your body on the fast track to maximizing fat loss for the rest of the day.

DAY 2 ▶
INCREASE YOUR AWARENESS

Let us not look back in anger or forward in fear, but around in awareness.
— JAMES THURBER

All change begins with awareness. If, for example, a ship is off course, it isn't until the captain becomes aware of the problem that he is able to make a correction.

To see how that works, spend the day observing other people. Without judging, observe how they eat, listen closely to what they say, become more aware of the differences in behavior between those who are overweight and those who are not. Do you think the people you are observing are aware of how they appear to you?

Now, enlist the support of someone who has known you for a while. (Your best choice for a confidant may not necessarily be your closest relative or spouse.) Tell the person that you are starting on a new approach to getting in shape, and you need to ask five questions, for which you need honest responses.

Ask the following questions in the order given:

1. I am in the process of losing weight. Did you realize that I needed to lose a few pounds?
2. How long do you think I have wanted to lose weight?
3. In your opinion, what would you say is the reason I'm overweight?
4. What do you think is going to be my biggest challenge in losing weight and keeping it off?
5. When it comes to nutrition, exercise, or attitude in regard to losing weight, which do you think is my biggest strength, and why?

Write the answers in your journal and note how you felt about the answers. We'll be revisiting these questions and answers at the end of 21 days.

▶ Fresh Start Reminder

HEIGHTENING YOUR AWARENESS by journaling everything you eat, the time you eat it, and your mood and thoughts is the easiest way to double your fat loss.

DAY 3 ▶
GET MOTIVATED NOW!

Prepare your mind to receive the best that life has to offer.
—ERNEST HOLMES

I know you want to lose weight. And guess what? You are going to do it! As a matter of fact, you are already doing it. Today I want you to come up with a motive that's strong enough to keep you going. You probably recall that we talked about the importance of finding your true motivation in Chapter 2.

When I ask clients to tell me what's motivating them to lose weight, their answers are often along the lines of, "So that I can be around for my children or grandchildren." That sounds good, but when I then ask, "Are you able to be with your children or grandchildren *now*?" they almost always say yes. This is an example of how even the most sincere reason may not always be strong enough to move you to take action. Here's why: When you can be with your children or grandchildren *now*, the motive isn't strong enough. What you're really saying is that *if* at some time in the future you couldn't be with your children or grandchildren because of your weight-related health issues, then and only then would you do something.

We humans are very shortsighted and have a hard time accepting delayed gratification. While big-picture motives are admirable and essential, more often than not we can't sustain any action, whether it's saving money, planning a trip, or getting in shape, without an immediate incentive—a motive that resonates with us *right now*, not next month or next year or in 10 years.

Connecting a reason with a decision to take action is how we come to *motivation*.

▶ Fresh Start Reminder

WHEN YOU KNOW *why* you are doing what you do, you are more likely to carry through to your goal. Therefore, getting and staying motivated is fueled by gathering information that supports your healthful habits.

DAY 4 ▶
SET A REALISTIC GOAL FOR YOURSELF

The future you see is the future you get.
—ROBERT G. ALLEN

Your task for today is to set a realistic goal for where you will be at the end of 21 days. I suggest that you make it your mission (after your first week of losing up to 7 pounds) to continue to lose from 1 to 3 pounds a week. If you lose more, that's great, but it's more important to set a goal that's achievable. To remind yourself of why that's so important, you can go back and reread Chapter 5.

Having a short-term goal, such as losing 1 to 3 pounds a week, helps you remain enthusiastic about each day. Throughout our lives, we are practically programmed to be goal oriented. As we go through elementary school, our goal is to get promoted each year. Then, in high school, our goal is to graduate and move on to college or a career. As we enter the working world, we set goals for moving up the corporate ladder or building a business. Having a goal is what keeps us engaged and pulls us forward, whether it's having a family, running a marathon, getting a job promotion, or losing unwanted pounds.

Too many of us either don't have a goal or set goals that are unachievable. Either way, we sabotage our own chances for success. If we have no goal, we have no direction. If we set a goal that's beyond our capability, we're creating a formula for failure.

Once you've achieved your first weight loss goal, set a new one for the next 21 days. By continuing to reset your realistic goals, you will continue to succeed. The moment you take your eye off the ball and announce to yourself that you don't need a new goal, you are likely to end up either gaining the weight back or failing to make any progress.

▶ Fresh Start Reminder

EXPERIMENTING WITH DIFFERENT varieties of fat-burning meals will help you avoid the boredom so often associated with failed diets. You can find many combinations to choose from in Chapter 6. And for inspiration, try some of the recipes in Chapter 11.

DAY 5 ▶
IT'S YOUR CHOICE

It's choice—not chance—that determines your destiny.
—JEAN NIDETCH, FOUNDER OF WEIGHT WATCHERS

Just because you want something doesn't mean you automatically choose it. I may *want* to eat a whole pizza all at once, but I *choose* not to do so. It would be nice to eat a whole pizza and not have to contend with the consequences of my action, but that isn't a realistic possibility.

You may think that you don't always have a choice, but that isn't true either. Take work for example. You may think that you don't have a choice about going to work, but you do. You choose to go to work to earn money, pay for groceries and electricity, and clothe yourself and your family. You could also choose not to go to work, which would mean choosing not to earn money, not to pay the grocery and electric bills, and not to buy clothes for yourself and your family. If you get a traffic ticket, you have a choice to pay it or not. When you pay it, you are making the choice to avoid a penalty, which saves you money and keeps you out of jail.

There's always a choice, and the choice you make always has consequences. To have a diet-free mindset is to understand that you truly have a choice every moment of every day. In the words of Albert Camus, "Life is the sum of all your choices."

Today I want you to write in your journal three choices you have made that reinforce your desire to live diet-free. These choices might be as simple as deciding to switch from sugary sodas to sugar-free drinks (even to water) or to carry healthful snacks to eat during the day or to start off the day with a good breakfast. Your choices, like your goals and motivations, don't have to be monumental and earth shattering—but they will be life changing.

▶ Fresh Start Reminder

WHEN YOU CHOOSE to combine fast and slow carbs in the proper proportions, you are choosing to maximize fat burning and be lean and healthy.

DAY 6 ▶
LEARN THE DIFFERENCE BETWEEN THINKING AND FEELING

> Gluttony is an emotional escape, a sign something is eating us.
> —PETER DE VRIES

Someone says something hurtful or offensive, and without thinking, you respond in a way that isn't very nice. When that happens, you're responding without thinking. And when life is tossing bricks at you, it's easy to be led by your emotions. Today you might be doing everything right. Tomorrow you get upset and soothe yourself by turning to food. Some therapists refer to this as self-medicating with food in response to an emotional disturbance. Others believe that it's a way to take your mind off your problem.

Whatever you call it, when you're in the throes of an emotional situation, it can be challenging to tap into your core motivation and choose to eat in a way that supports your decision to be diet-free. I'm not saying that emotions are bad; they're what make our life worth living. The key, however, is not to let them get in the way of rational thinking.

When I was a youngster, my grandmother encouraged me to walk away from upsetting situations, take a few deep breaths, and count to 10. I could avoid being led by my emotions into doing something I would later regret. Instead, I could calm down and cope with the situation rationally.

When it comes to making decisions about food, the goal is to be led by your thoughts, not your emotions. Now determine how you could have responded in a more rational way to each of those situations. The more aware you become of the difference between thinking and feeling, the less likely you'll be to allow your emotions to take control of your actions.

▶ Fresh Start Reminder

WHEN YOU PLAN your meals and snacks in advance, you are more likely to make thoughtful rather than emotional decisions about what and how much you eat.

DAY 7 ▶
NEVER GIVE UP

> Obstacles don't have to stop you. If you run into a wall,
> don't turn around and give up. Figure out how to climb it,
> go through it, or work around it.
> —MICHAEL JORDAN

You have made a decision to move forward, shed inches, and drop pounds, but I'm sure you have had one, two, or more thoughts enter your mind that aren't supportive of your decision. When we make a decision to improve any part of our life, opposition and obstacles will show up. Adversity is a part of life, but it doesn't have to stop you from achieving your goal.

Today, take 15 minutes to think about what obstacles you are likely to face as you follow your intention to live a diet-free life. If you're having a difficult time coming up with potential challenges or difficulties, look at the fourth question you asked your friend on Day 2: *What do you think is going to be my biggest challenge in losing weight and keeping it off?* What was your friend's answer to that question? Do you agree? If not, what other challenges do you think will be even bigger? Still having trouble? Revisit the possible obstacles I listed in Chapter 4.

Once you've identified your own personal roadblocks, write down *two* things you could do to get around each one. If your motivation for achieving your goal is strong enough, you can figure out a way to overcome any obstacle.

From now on, whenever you have a negative or discouraging thought or find yourself in a situation that could be leading you off track, write it down. Then come up with two ideas for how you can avoid or overcome it in the future.

▶ Fresh Start Reminder

NOTICE YOUR ENERGY levels after you snack. If your snack isn't giving you the energy you need, try something higher in carbohydrates. Eating a snack that's higher in protein than carbs may not be providing enough carbs to keep your blood sugar level from dropping too low.

AFTER 7 DAYS, STOP AND REASSESS

At this point you've probably noticed that your clothes are a bit looser and you are feeling more energetic, less sluggish, and mentally and physically *lighter*! So, let's see how your fat loss is progressing.

Time for Another Photo

First, take another set of photos. I suggest that you wear the same thing you wore when you took the "before" pictures a week ago. I'm sure you've been looking in the mirror, but as I've said, it's easy to forget what you looked like before. When you put those two sets of photos side by side, you'll be able to see how much progress you've made in such a short time.

Weigh In

Get back on the scale and see where you now stand in terms of total weight, fat weight, and lean body mass. Remember, if you used a Tanita scale or another method to establish a baseline for your weight and percentage of body fat, use the same scale or method now, and be sure to weigh yourself at about the same time of day. Check the numbers against the ones you recorded a week ago. Whether or not your total weight has already changed, you should see a shift in your body composition toward a higher percentage of lean muscle and a lower percentage of fat.

Remeasure

Redo the measurements I asked you to take in Chapter 4. Record them in your journal next to your pre–fat loss measurements and see how the numbers have changed. Even if you haven't lost pounds, you should be losing inches. If you've lost inches—whatever your body fat percentage or scale weight—you are smaller, and that is worth celebrating. Your body has improved, and you have a new baseline. Whether your weight has dropped or your inches are reduced or both, if you continue doing what you've been doing, the numbers will fall into place.

I know I said that when you live diet-free, you could expect to lose *up to 7* pounds and 7 inches in 7 days; I didn't say that everyone of you would *absolutely* lose that much. Remember the client I told you about who was discouraged because she'd lost *only* 5 pounds in 3 weeks? Her expectations were unrealistic, and she needed to understand that this was not a short-term crash diet but the beginning of a new way of life.

How much change you are seeing at the end of this first week is largely determined by where you were when you started. If you are content with the changes you see, keep on doing exactly what you have been doing. If you would like to see more change more quickly, now is the time to reassess and make a few more changes as you move forward.

Where You Might Go Wrong

1. **Not eating often enough.** Are you eating every 2 to 3 hours up to 1 hour before you go to sleep? If not, you may be encouraging your metabolism to slow down and letting your blood sugar drop too low so that your body is more prone to store fat.
2. **Exercising less.** If you were already exercising, have you stopped completely or exercised less often for some reason? If so, you may have lost some lean body mass and consequently slowed your metabolic rate. Remember, muscle burns calories more quickly than fat does. Getting back to your regular routine should solve this problem.
3. **Eating and exercise.** If you exercise, are you eating at the proper intervals before and after your workout? Except when doing light cardio first thing in the morning, are you eating a snack before and a meal or a snack within an hour after your workout? If you're not sure you're doing this correctly, review Chapter 7 for my eating and exercise guide.
4. **Not eating enough protein.** When you eat a meal, you need to be sure that it includes the right quantity of protein. Protein slows down the rate at which carbs are metabolized and, therefore, helps your body maximize fat loss and keeps your blood sugar from spiking too high. If you've been getting enough protein at meal times, take a look at your snacks. If most of your snacks are primarily carbs (like an apple), consider replacing one with something (such as an energy bar) that has at least 10 grams of protein. I know I said that you could snack on just about anything as long as it didn't

Q What is the best snack to have in the morning before my major workout? I run 13 to 15 miles. I have been having a banana. —Amy P. (Milwaukee, WI)

A To make the most of your workout and maximize fat burning, when you are performing a high-intensity workout like resistance training or an endurance workout like running 13 to 15 miles, it is best either to eat a meal or to have a snack about an hour before. But whether it's a meal or a snack, make sure that what you're eating has carbs—specifically those that are highest in glucose or starch, such as a banana, oatmeal, or a Clif or Luna energy bar. And be sure you have a meal within 30 to 60 minutes of completing your exercise session. For more carb recommendations that are highest in glucose, go to www.dietfreelife.com.

FAQ

exceed the recommended number of calories, and there is certainly nothing wrong with an apple. But everyone's body is different, and some of us require more protein than others—particularly if we are exercising regularly.

5. **Not eating enough carbohydrates.** Many of my clients are surprised to learn that when we don't eat enough carbohydrates during the course of the day, we are likely to see a drop in our lean body mass, which results in an increase in body fat. Carbohydrates are the primary source of fuel for your body and your brain, and when your body isn't getting enough fuel, you are less likely to maximize your fat-burning potential. Review your carb intake during your meal and especially following your workouts. I recommend that you consume *no fewer than* 30 grams of carbohydrates at every meal. If you know you are getting adequate amounts of carbs in your meals, revisit your snacks. In my experience, people often go from one extreme to the other when it is the proper balance of nutrients that is actually the key to fat loss.

6. **Not eating enough calories.** If you have lost weight but your percentage of fat has increased with relation to your lean body mass, you've probably been eating too little. Your body thinks there's a famine coming and is thus starting to store fat instead of burning it. While I'm not an advocate of long-term calorie counting, I

suggest that you track your calories for a week or two and make sure you are consuming enough—1,200 a day for women and 1,500 for men. The best way to add calories is to increase your protein intake until you see your percentage of body fat begin to drop.

7. **Eating too many calories.** If you have gained weight and haven't lost inches, you are eating too much food for your body weight and activity level. If this is the case, I recommend you consider counting your calories for a couple of weeks so that you can track down and eliminate the excess calories that may have been sneaking into your daily intake without your being aware of them. When you do this, you will discover how much of an impact a few little tweaks can have on your ability to drop pounds quickly.

8. **Not drinking enough water.** How much water are you drinking? Your muscles are more than 70 percent water, and since muscle is primarily responsible for your body being able to burn fat, it is to your benefit to keep your muscles hydrated so that they burn fat more efficiently. I recommend that you work your way up to 8 to 12 (8-ounce) glasses of water, and add an additional 8-ounce glass for every 20 minutes of exercise you do. Also, if you live in an area where it is humid, drink more water. Finally, although this may seem paradoxical, the more water you drink, the less likely you are to retain water. The last thing you want is to do everything right and still see your total body weight increase because you are retaining water.

Revisit Your Personal Metabolism Profile Quiz

You have taken the quiz, tallied your results, and figured out where you need to make changes. Now you can go back and take another look at the areas where you need the most improvement.

- Have you been eating breakfast within 30 to 60 minutes of waking up every day?
- Have you been eating a meal or snacking every 2 to 3 hours?
- Have you been combining your preferred foods in a way that encourages fat burning?
- Have you been eating fast and slow carbs in the right combinations and proportions?

- Have you kept your intake of fat to the suggested amounts and increased the quantity of lean protein in your diet?
- Have you cut down on fat condiments so that you are less likely to exceed the recommended amounts?
- Could you do more exercise to get rid of that fat around your middle?
- Are you drinking too much alcohol and not enough water?
- Are you getting enough sleep?
- Are you eating more than the recommended amount of fast carbs?
- What kinds of snacks are you eating most often?
- Are you eating a preworkout snack when performing resistance training or high-intensity cardio?
- Have you been eating a meal within 60 minutes of completing your workouts?

As you continue to make adjustments, don't try to change everything at once. If you do that, it may be too overwhelming, and you will be more likely to quit—the same way you might have quit the diets you have been on in the past.

DAY 8 ▶
GET MOVING

> Exercise is king, nutrition is queen, but together you have the entire kingdom.
>
> — JACK LALANNE

On the first day of the second week of your makeover, you're going to step it up by integrating some exercise into your life. If you're already working out on a regular basis, that's great. However, many of my clients start to roll their eyes and groan at the very mention of the word *exercise*. If you're like them, you've probably tried it, had an unpleasant experience, and quit. That's why I'm going to meet you where you are right now.

You can start by staying in motion for no more than 12 minutes at a time 3 days a week and still achieve results. And you can fit those 12 minutes into your schedule any way you want. Take a brisk walk in the morning, go to the gym at lunchtime, or pop in a DVD and work out at home in the evening. You can do that!

Read Chapter 10 and learn about the CircuFit program to determine what's going to work for you based on your current fitness and your exercise history. Keep it real, and don't get so ambitious that you set yourself up for failure. You need to figure out how often and how long you can *realistically* exercise each week.

Finally, as you move forward with your fitness, keep in mind these wise words from former heavyweight boxing champ Muhammad Ali: "Champions aren't made in gyms. Champions are made from something they have deep inside them—a desire, a dream, a vision. They have to have last-minute stamina, they have to be a little faster, and they have to have the skill and the will. But the will must be stronger than the skill."

I know you have the will. You are a champion!

▶ Fresh Start Reminder

THE MOST DIFFICULT part of fitness is getting it done. If you haven't been able to fit exercise into your routine, consider starting your day 15 to 30 minutes earlier. Remember, it takes only 12 minutes a day to start getting fit.

DAY 9 ▶
GIVE YOURSELF PERMISSION TO FALL FORWARD

> Our greatest glory lies not in never falling but in rising every time we fall.
> — CONFUCIUS

If you're afraid of falling (or failing), you may never begin, which means that you're more or less guaranteed not to succeed. Think about the toddler learning to walk. At first he falls every time he takes a step, but he gets back up and tries again, and eventually he's walking without falling.

The first 8 days of your diet-free life probably weren't perfect. No one is expected to be perfect the first time he or she attempts anything new. You've no doubt come up against a few obstacles you hadn't anticipated, and those may have made you doubt yourself. But there's always a way around an obstacle, so the next time you find yourself blindsided by an unexpected roadblock, go back to Day 7 and come up with two tactics for getting around it in the future. When you approach an obstacle that way, it becomes a learning experience, and every learning experience leaves you better, not worse, off. Each time you learn from a mistake, you're falling forward, and you wind up further down the road to a diet-free life than you were before you fell.

Today, start to change the way you think about falling. Falling is different from failing, and so long as you keep getting up and trying again, you haven't failed. In fact, you've made progress. The only way to fail is to stop trying—or never to have tried at all. So, take a moment on this day to applaud yourself for having fallen, and give yourself a pat on the back for getting up and moving on.

▶ Fresh Start Reminder

ALWAYS REMEMBER TO eat a meal or a snack within an hour after you finish exercising. For more on eating and exercise, see Chapter 7.

DAY 10 ▶
OVERCOME TEMPTATION WITH MENTAL REHEARSAL

> The strangest secret is that we become what we think about, most of the time.
> —EARL NIGHTINGALE

Temptation is one of the biggest obstacles when trying to lose weight. That's when having a diet-free mindset can really come to the rescue, and the best way to reinforce that mindset is through mental rehearsal.

Not long ago I was having breakfast with my friend Art. Partway through the meal, he offered me half his biscuit, and I declined. "Come on," he insisted, "try it. It's really good." I said no again. "Just take a bite," he pushed. "No one's looking." When I refused again, he let it go.

As we were leaving the restaurant, I asked Art why he'd been so insistent. At first he said he'd just wanted me to taste it because it was so good. But when I asked why he'd continued to push me after I'd said no, he admitted that he didn't want to eat the whole thing and thought he'd feel better about eating it if I shared it.

When you're in the presence of a food pusher or at an event where temptation is all around you it can be really hard to stick with your healthier choices. But you can use the same strategy elite athletes do when preparing for a competition: They *mentally rehearse* their game plan.

Take a few minutes to imagine that you're having dinner with a food pusher like Art, and mentally practice how you're going to respond. Visualize the event from start to finish, and see yourself saying no to temptation.

Just as your muscles benefit from regular exercise, so does your mind. The more often you take time to visualize yourself performing a certain way, the more likely you will be to manifest that behavior in reality.

▶ Fresh Start Reminder

WHEN YOU GO to a restaurant, mentally rehearse in advance what you're going to order to create your fat-burning meal. If you need help, revisit the tips for dining out in Chapter 7.

DAY 11 ▶
BOLSTER YOUR MOTIVATION WITH KNOWLEDGE

Zeal without knowledge is fire without light.
—THOMAS FULLER

One of the main reasons people aren't able to sustain their motivation and experience lasting success after losing weight is because they don't really understand *why* they're doing what they're doing—and why it's actually working.

I know when you took this book home you were eager to get started, and you may very well have skipped over the chapters explaining how your biology and body composition respond to nutrition and exercise. Today, go back and read (or reread) Chapter 3 carefully so that you really understand how blood sugar relates to fat burning.

Even little kids want to know why they need to do something. Do you remember how you responded when your mother asked you to do something? More often than not you probably asked, "Why? Why do I have to?" As adults, we still want to know why. That knowledge is what keeps us motivated to continue.

If you're just following any weight loss or exercise guidelines without understanding the reasoning behind them, you might find yourself succumbing to the promise of the next big diet fad even if you've been having a measure of success already. If you're really committed to changing your mindset so that living diet-free becomes your way of life, you need to understand why you're doing the things you do.

▶ Fresh Start Reminder

IF YOU'VE BEEN doing the same exercise routine over and over, try changing it up so that your body doesn't get used to doing the same movement all the time. Doing something different will increase the return you see on your exercise investment. The more you know about how your body reacts to different kinds of exercise, the better able you'll be to exercise efficiently. Read Chapter 10 to learn how to maximize your fitness.

DAY 12 ▶
DEFINE THE ACTIONS THAT WILL GET YOU TO YOUR GOAL

Our goals can only be reached through the vehicle of a plan, in which we must fervently believe, and upon which we must vigorously act.
—STEPHEN A. BRENNAN

On Day 4, I asked you to set a realistic goal for where you want to be in terms of your weight and fitness at the end of 21 days. Today, take some time to articulate the actions that will help you get there. I'm sure that you've already been making changes in the way you eat and how often you exercise, but you may not have been acknowledging those changes clearly to yourself. So, in your journal, write down five specific actions that are going to help maximize your fat loss. These actions might be making sure to eat every 2 to 3 hours or to drink 12 (8-ounce) glasses of water a day. A third might be exercising for at least 12 minutes 3 days a week. Writing down these action steps makes them concrete and clarifies them in your mind.

Get in the habit of doing this every night before you go to bed. Without looking at the ones you wrote on previous days, make a list of five actions. Sometimes you may find that you repeat steps, but it is all in aid of reinforcing your ultimate goal. When on Day 21 you review all the actions you wrote down, you'll be surprised to see how they've evolved in the course of the 10 days you've been doing this and how many of them have already become so much a part of your new mindset that you do them unconsciously.

▶ Fresh Start Reminder

AS YOUR FITNESS level increases, remember to step up your exercise so that you continue to maximize fat loss. Look at Chapter 10 to see whether it's time to move up to the next level.

DAY 13 ▶
LEARN NOT TO JUDGE YOURSELF

> Striving for excellence motivates you; striving for perfection is demoralizing.
>
> —HARRIET BRAIKER

As you move toward living diet-free, there will be many opportunities for you to judge yourself—and find yourself lacking. Doing that is one of the quickest ways to put out your motivational fire.

On Day 9, you started thinking of mistakes as opportunities to learn. Now, it's time to stop judging yourself against some self-imposed standard you think you should be meeting. Self-judgment just leads to guilt, and guilt leads to negativity.

Maybe you ate something that wasn't in your meal plan for the day and now you're beating yourself up about it. Or perhaps you missed a session at the gym. Despite our best-laid plans, we all mess up now and then.

Today, stop and think about the last time you judged yourself harshly. How did that make you feel? There's no value to be had in putting yourself down. Instead, take another look at what you did (or didn't do) that caused you to think so badly of yourself, and determine the reason for your perceived failure. If you can figure out *why* the situation occurred, it will become a valuable lesson instead of a liability.

Now, show yourself the kind of compassion you'd like others to show you. Tell yourself what you'd tell your dearest friend in the same situation. Then forgive yourself for not being perfect—and move on.

▶ Fresh Start Reminder

MAKE THE EFFORT to choose leaner protein sources—such as chicken and turkey breasts or nonfatty fish, including halibut or tilapia—more often than fattier proteins. The leaner your protein, the less saturated fat you'll consume and the more you'll be maximizing fat loss.

DAY 14 ▶
PUT A POSITIVE SPIN ON YOUR FUTURE

Once you replace negative thoughts with positive ones,
you'll start having positive results.
—WILLIE NELSON

How is your life going to be improved when you reach your weight loss goal? What in your life is going to be better compared to where you are right now?

I've posed these questions thousands of times—to clients, to people I've met at the local café, and even to those sitting in a doctor's waiting room. What amazes me is how often the answers I receive are put in negative terms. *I won't have to shop in the plus-size department anymore. I won't have people staring at me when I'm shopping in the supermarket. I won't have to feel guilty about taking up so much room on the bus.*

Isn't the point of being diet-free to have a *better* life than you do now? The only way to make that happen is to change the way you think about your future. Today, go back and review the value of positive self-talk in Chapter 2.

Think about how many times you've told yourself what *won't* happen when you've dropped the fat, and see how many times you can reword those statements so that they reflect what *will* happen. *I'll be able to buy all those cute clothes my friends are always wearing. I'll be so proud of myself as I check out with all my weight loss foods at the supermarket. I'll feel great as I slide into that tiny seat on the bus.*

Remember, positive self-talk leads to positive outcomes.

▶ Fresh Start Reminder

IT'S DAY 14—TIME to take a new measure of yourself. If you want to step up your progress in the next 7 days, try eating snacks that are closer to 100 calories than 200 or 300. These little tweaks can make a big difference.

DAY 15 ▶
DEBUNK THE DIET LIES

The naked truth is always better than the best dressed lie.
—ANN LANDERS

Can you lose weight by avoiding foods like bread, potatoes, and cereal? Can you lose weight on a plan that awards points to everything you put in your mouth? Can you lose weight eating only prepackaged meals? The answer to all these questions is yes. When you set your mind to stick to a diet, no matter what kind it is, you will lose weight. The real question is whether you have to endure that kind of deprivation to lose weight and whether you can live with that kind of restriction forever.

Almost every one of my clients has lost weight before on one kind of diet or another. And almost every one of those diets is based on the lie that it is the *only* way to win at weight loss. You've probably been on one or more of those diets yourself. Make a list of the different diets you've been on. Then write down the lie on which each of them was based. For example: To lose weight, you must give up eating carbohydrates. But if you've been following the Diet-Free for Life approach, you've been eating potatoes, pasta, and cereal and still dropping pounds and gaining lean muscle tissue.

Recognizing and debunking those diet lies and false promises will reinforce your mindset and ensure that you no longer fall prey to the diet mentality.

▶ Fresh Start Reminder

YOU NEED TO eat carbohydrates to keep your blood sugar from dropping too low. It's the way that you combine fast and slow carbs and what you eat with them that helps you maximize fat loss, not avoiding them completely. In fact, not eating carbs is counterproductive when you're living diet-free.

DAY 16 ▶
OWN WHAT YOU KNOW

In a time of turbulence and change, it is more true than ever that knowledge is power.
—JOHN F. KENNEDY

Some of the concepts in this book may contradict what you've been told all your life about weight loss. But in the past 2 weeks or so, you've learned a great deal. In fact, you may be surprised by how much you know. Take a few minutes to write down all the things you now know about fat loss that you didn't know when you started to make over your mind and body.

Knowing goes a step beyond thinking. If you *think* you know the answer to something, it's possible that you are unsure or that you'll still change your mind. If you *know* it, you've really embraced the truth of your thoughts. Knowing powers doing. When you *know* something to be true, you're much more likely to act on it than if you only *think* it might be true.

If I woke up tomorrow and discovered that I'd somehow become heavier, I'd be momentarily frustrated or even alarmed. But then I'd quickly calm down because I know without question how to eat and exercise in a way that will quickly get that weight off. And now, so do you. Once you really own what you know, nothing and no one will be able to dissuade you; you will no longer have any doubts about what you need to do.

▶ Fresh Start Reminder

IF YOU HAVEN'T already done so, now is the time to reweigh and remeasure yourself. Looking at the changes you've made will help reinforce the fact that you now really do *know* how to live diet-free.

DAY 17 ▶
MAKE WEIGHT LOSS A TOP PRIORITY

A major part of successful living lies in the ability to put first things first.

—STEVEN R. COVEY

You're really motivated, and you know how your life is going to improve when you have lost weight, have gotten fit, and are living diet-free. But then somehow life gets in the way and you let things slide. It happens. We all have so many things competing for our time and attention.

You know what to do: You know how to make a fat-burning meal, you know how to snack, you know how to exercise, and really, it's not that difficult. If you aren't doing everything you can to achieve your goal, you must have other priorities that are higher on your list. Even if you're motivated, until weight loss becomes a top priority, you're not going to give it all you've got.

To help you get on the fast track, I challenge you to write out a to-do list with at least 10 things on it. Where does weight loss come on that list? If it's number 10 or even number 6, there's a good chance you're not going to be paying enough attention. What you need to do is reset your priorities so that dropping pounds and inches is number 1. You have to eat every day, so why not do it in the healthiest, most beneficial way you can. Make fat loss *numero uno*, and you're sure to get to it!

▶ Fresh Start Reminder

IN THE MIDST of your busy day, don't forget to snack. Have a piece of chocolate in the afternoon or after dinner. Just be sure the chocolate you choose is higher in fat calories than in sugar and carbs. (Remember that a portion of chocolate is 1 ounce for women and 1 to 2 ounces for men.)

DAY 18 ▶
LEARN TO THINK DIET-FREE

I'm living my life, not buying a lifestyle.
— BARBARA KRUGER

Being diet-free means living your life by choosing to eat in a way that supports your unique circumstances. In fact, the word *diet* has been corrupted in recent years to mean something different from its original definition. If you begin to think of a diet as the sum total of the foods you eat on a regular basis, you'll actually be thinking diet-free.

If you were gluten sensitive, you'd be avoiding foods that contain wheat. If you're lactose intolerant, you avoid milk products. Vegetarians don't eat meat. People who are kosher don't eat shellfish. Those with peanut allergies stay away from peanuts. These aren't temporary solutions; they're choices people make so that they can live healthier and happier *throughout their lives.*

Make a list of all the food and beverage choices you make that aren't temporary and aren't related to weight loss. When you have that list in front of you, it will be easier for you to understand that deciding what foods you're going to eat and how you're going to eat them is just one of the many choices we make every day about how to live our life.

Living diet-free means that you've decided never again to succumb to the mentality that says "going on a diet" is going to provide a permanent solution to your lifelong battle with weight.

▶ Fresh Start Reminder

WHEN EATING IN a restaurant, remember that the menu is written on paper, not in stone. You can ask for your meal to be prepared in a way that supports your decision to remain diet-free. After all, you'd do that if you had a food allergy, wouldn't you?

DAY 19 ▶
LEARN WHAT YOU CAN AND CANNOT CHANGE

> Everyone thinks of changing the world, but no one thinks
> of changing himself.
> — LEO TOLSTOY

It's time to come to grips with the fact that the only person you can change is *you*. You cannot change other people's feelings or behaviors, and once you accept that, you'll be better able to keep your mind on doing for yourself what no one else can do for you. To maximize fat loss, the only person you need to win over is you. It would certainly be nice to have the support of your friends and family, but that doesn't always happen, and there's not much you can do to make it happen. So you need to be your own support system.

As much as you may want the people close to you to eat the way you do, they may not be ready to make that change. It's a decision they're each going to have to make for themselves in their own time. You don't want them to think less of you for your choice, so try not to judge them for theirs.

Many people decide to lose weight because they believe it will make someone else—a spouse, a lover, or a family member—think better of them. Maybe it will, but then again, maybe it won't. You can't change the way someone else thinks about you, so you need to create the changes that will make you think better of yourself.

Go back to the list you made on Day 14 of the ways your life would be different if you lost weight. Did any of your answers involve changing the way other people thought or felt about you? If so, see if you can revise those responses to make them all about you.

▶ Fresh Start Reminder

WHEN YOU'RE WORKING out, avoid comparing yourself with others. Fitness needs to start with where you are in terms of health and ability—not with the person on the treadmill beside you.

DAY 20 ▶
LEARN TO LIVE WITH IMPERFECTION

> Have no fear of perfection—you'll never reach it.
> — SALVADOR DALÍ

I can't tell you how many clients walk into my clinic and, before I can even say hello, announce how bad they were with their eating over the weekend.

As you near the last day of your 21-Day Mindset Makeover, understand that you'll never meet a person who is perfect—*never*—and that includes you. If you can just accept the fact that you're not perfect, you'll be saving yourself a lot of heartache. Go back and revisit what you learned on Days 9 and 13. Remind yourself that with every mistake you make, you're learning something new, and renew your decision to stop judging yourself harshly.

To reinforce those choices, be constantly on guard about thinking negatively about yourself, and immediately turn that negative thought into a positive. If, for example, you find yourself thinking, "I'm so stupid; I should have known better," turn that around so that you're saying, "I really learned something today. It's going to make me smarter from now on."

What you do is always a manifestation of how you think.

▶ Fresh Start Reminder

CONTINUING TO FINE-TUNE your decisions about food and exercise will enhance your fat loss. Go back and read Chapters 3 and 10 to see what you might want to change. In living diet-free, as in everything about life, there's always room to do better.

DAY 21 ▶
FOLLOW UP AND FOLLOW THROUGH

> I can give you a six-word formula for success: Think things
> through—then follow through.
> —EDDIE RICKENBACKER

You have reached the 21-day milestone and should have now made living diet-free your new way of looking at your life. To show you how far you've come, I want you to go back and revisit the questions you asked your friend on Day 2.

1. *I am in the process of losing weight. Did you realize that I needed to lose a few pounds?*
   Do you feel differently about your friend's answer now than you did when you first asked the question? Do you think he or she would answer it the same way today?

2. *How long do you think I have wanted to lose weight?*
   Was your friend right? Were you aware of how long you'd wanted to do this without actually putting your wishes into action? Is there one thing you can name as the catalyst that finally got you started?

3. *In your opinion, what would you say is the reason or reasons I'm overweight?*
   Do you think your friend had a realistic image of you? Did the answer you got help you to become more self-aware? How have you changed the way you approach the issues or habits that caused you to gain weight in the past?

4. *What do you think is going to be my biggest challenge in losing weight and keeping it off?*
   Was your friend right, or have you found some other challenge more difficult to handle? How has the 21-Day Mindset Makeover helped you cope with your challenges?

5. *When it comes to nutrition, exercise, or attitude in regard to losing weight, which do you think is my biggest strength, and why?*
Again, did it turn out that your friend was correct? What have you found to be your greatest strength, and why?

As you review the answers you got and the ones you're now giving, do you see how much your approach to food and fitness has already evolved? Now, make another call to the person you spoke with at the beginning of this process and see if his or her answers have changed. While your assessment of your progress should never be based on someone else's opinion, it's possible that he or she will see changes in you that you yourself have missed.

▶ **Fresh Start Reminder**

YOU ARE A work in progress, so please continue to review the steps you've taken to help you reinforce and readjust your thoughts as you continue to move forward.

10

Step It Up:
Start to Exercise

I believe that exercise has been given too much credit for increasing a person's ability to lose weight. It is something I personally enjoy, and I certainly encourage everyone to exercise because it has great health benefits. But when it comes to fat loss, exercise, in and of itself, is not the answer. That said, however, increasing physical activity can certainly speed up the process. And regular exercise will also make it possible for you to eat more once you've arrived at your goal weight because you'll be burning fat more efficiently.

From giving you more energy to getting you more fit, exercise, combined with proper nutrition, allows you to lose fat faster. Just ask Freddi G., who attended my Fit Camp. Freddi simply needed a little push to get started with his fitness program. Well, that is what he thought at first. What he quickly discovered is that to truly transform one's body, it is essential to upgrade not only one's fitness but also one's nutrition and mindset.

In the past, he believed that in order to lean out, he needed to exercise between 2 and 3 hours a day. Freddi did not have this kind of time. However, with my multimuscle matrix approach to getting a total body workout in a limited time—a workout that could be performed at home or anywhere for that matter—Freddi was able to fit exercise into his schedule.

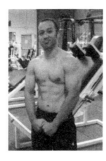

While implementing the Fresh Start and the CircuFit workouts into his schedule, Freddi G. dropped 10 pounds the first 21 days. Starting at 214 pounds and considered obese (body fat percentage of 28), Freddi leaned out, and in less than 4 months, he weighed in at 154 pounds with 8.3 percent body fat.

The problem, as I see it, is that far too many people are exercising furiously without substantially reducing their waistline. As reporter John Cloud pointed out in his 2009 *Time* magazine article titled "Why Exercise Won't Make You Thin": "More than 45 million Americans now belong to a health club, up from 23 million in 1993." And, he continued, "We spend some $19 billion a year on gym memberships." This is no surprise to me, because week after week I meet people who begin our conversation by letting me know how frustrated they are that the weight isn't coming off even though they're spending more and more time at the gym. Then, when I mention nutrition to these gym goers, they are quick to let me know that they're eating healthy, so there must be something wrong with their metabolism or hormones or something else that is beyond their control.

The real reason, however, is this: We live in a society that tells us that if we want to make more money, we need to work more hours. We've been taught to believe that the more time we put in, the more money we'll make, and we've transferred that belief to our approach to exercise. We think that the more we work out, the more we sweat, the better the results. But the fact is, in terms of both work and working out, we need to do it smarter, not longer. We need to upgrade the quality of our work and our workouts, not the quantity.

Pam A. is a client who began going to a spinning class (indoor stationary cycling) and fell in love with it. She loved the music, the sweat, and the camaraderie. In the first 5 weeks she lost 10 pounds, and then the weight loss stopped. Pam couldn't understand why her body was no longer responding to her intense exercising, so I explained that if she wanted to keep losing weight, she would need to spin even longer and faster. But that wasn't her only problem. Weight-bearing activity—walking, running, kickboxing, or stepping, for example—is much more effective than non-weight-bearing activity for losing weight. Weight bearing is anything you do while supporting the weight of your own body.

When you're cycling, the bike is holding you up; if you're in the pool, the water is holding you up; and when you're on a rowing machine, the machine is holding you up. I have to add that if you are neither strong enough nor healthy enough to do weight-bearing exercise, it is important to start where you are—with non-weight-bearing activity—until you get strong enough to move on.

I told Pam she could keep on spinning but she'd have to change it up with some other kind of activity on alternate days. She still didn't believe me at first because she said, "I'm really sweating. You should see how much I sweat!" So I explained the concept of neuromuscular adaptation: for the first 3 to 5 weeks of performing a new activity, your body is working hard to adapt. Because what you're doing is new, you will see results. After that initial period, however, as your body adapts, you will need to either do *more* of that same activity or do something different to continue seeing the same results.

Then I suggested that for the next 2 weeks Pam make it a point to look at the other regular members of her class (not the beginners, because they would still be in the honeymoon period, when their bodies were adapting to the new activity) and see if she noticed any change in their bodies. She did that and reported back: "No one is getting smaller, Robert."

As I have shared with you throughout this book, nutrition is key, but so is the *quality* of your exercise. The kind of exercise I recommend is designed to maximize both short- and long-term results, and it will work for you no matter where you are at this moment in terms of overall fitness. So, if you are already exercising regularly and not seeing the results you would like, all I ask is that you keep an open mind and give my program a try. I won't ask you to spend endless hours working out. In fact, you may find that you are spending *less* time in the gym than you do now. And if you aren't yet working out, I will give you a program that meets you where you are now so that you can see and feel the changes, which will encourage you to continue and even step it up.

My mother is a good case in point. She is a breast cancer survivor who has two stents in her coronary arteries, has had both knees reconstructed, and has had a rotator cuff reconstructed twice. When she decided to become more active, she couldn't do any weight-bearing exercise, and I recommended that she find a fun fat-burning activity that would help her become more active.

Her fresh start to improved fitness was getting in the pool. She enrolled in a women-only health club and participated in its water-aerobics class. The goal was to build up her strength and endurance to the point where she would be able to do more. In less than 2 months, she began cross-training (that is, doing different types of exercise) by alternating her days in the pool with sessions on her stationary bike. In about 7 months, she had lost 50 pounds, felt lighter and stronger, and graduated to walking on a treadmill. At first she was able to walk for no more than 10 minutes without having to stop. She did this once and sometimes twice a week while continuing to use her stationary bike and do water aerobics.

As my mother got stronger, she was able to walk longer, she added an incline to her treadmill sessions, and the weight continued to come off. As I write this, she has lost more than 100 pounds and is able to walk on the treadmill for 60 minutes without stopping. The point I want to make here is that you need to start where you are because that is really the only place *to* start. And what helped my mom achieve her goal really comes down to her mindset. She set her intention to be able to do more, and she did.

When Stacy W. came to me, she was 47 years old, weighed almost 400 pounds, had 56 percent body fat, and hadn't exercised in years. We determined that based on her work schedule and other responsibilities, she would be able to get to the gym twice a week. I told her to start by getting on the treadmill and walking for 12 minutes without stopping, but I also told her that if she needed to take a break, she could do that.

At the end of the first week, Stacy called and told me that she had walked for 12 minutes without stopping both days and that she could have done more. "But," I told her, "I didn't want you to do more." Stacy didn't understand that, so I explained the concept of neuromuscular adaptation as I had to Pam, the spinning addict. I told her it was better for her to start slowly and build up gradually.

THE THREE PHASES OF EXERCISE

Before you begin to work out, it is important to understand that any exercise program has to include three phases: warm up, work out, and cool down.

There are a lot of people who don't think it's necessary to warm up. I see fit guys in the gym all the time who walk right over to the equipment and start working out without any warm-up at all. But the fact is, your muscles are primarily responsible for fat burning, and the longer you warm up, the more oxygen and blood there will be going to the working muscles, thereby maximizing the amount of fat you can burn both during and after your workout.

According to the American College of Sports Medicine, which sets the standard when it comes to exercise science, everyone should warm up for at least 6 to 12 minutes before a workout. And if you have a health issue such as shoulder or joint discomfort, I strongly recommend you take your time and warm up even longer—for up to 20 minutes.

Warming up means engaging in some kind of continuous movement, such as walking on a treadmill or performing the exercises you are going to be performing more slowly, which is referred to as an activity-specific warm-up. If you are extremely overweight or haven't done any kind of exercise since you were in high school, you may not be able to sustain continuous movement for more than 12 minutes, in which case those 12 minutes of walking may be your entire workout—and that is completely fine. You will still be burning fat, and as you increase your fitness, you will be able to do more and more.

Once you've completed your workout, you also need to cool down for at least 5 to 10 minutes. Cooling down allows your heart rate and breathing to return to normal levels gradually, so that you prevent blood pooling (major drops in blood pressure), which could lead to further complications (especially when the exerciser is unfit). Cooling down also prepares your muscles for your next exercise session and helps minimize the risk of muscle soreness after the workout. If you stop too abruptly after a vigorous workout, you could get dizzy or even faint. Worst-case scenario: You could actually have a heart attack. So make sure to take the necessary time to cool down at the end of your workout.

Choose the Program That's Right for You

In this chapter, I am going to give you two different 12-minute exercise programs I've used for years that progress from light cardio to high-intensity activity and work your entire body. In addition, depending on your level of fitness and the time you can put in, I'll provide you with a variety of weekly workout menus that range from 12 to 30 minutes in length (including the time it will take you to warm up and cool down).

These weekly plans are designed so that you alternate high-intensity with low-intensity workouts. It is important that you *do not* perform high-intensity exercises two days in a row because you need to give your muscles time to recover.

And finally, please bear in mind that these are recommendations designed to provide you with maximum results. If you find that you don't have the time to do 30 minutes on any given day, just 12 minutes of continuous activity will be enough to keep you on the fast track.

Figure Out Where You Are Now

Before you begin any kind of new exercise program, assess your present fitness level and determine whether you should first consult with your doctor by completing the following questionnaire.

Physical Activity Readiness Questionnaire

If you are between the ages of 15 and 69 and answer yes to any of the following questions, it is best that you talk with your doctor by phone or in person *before* you become more physically active and *before* you have a fitness appraisal. Tell your doctor about this questionnaire and the questions to which you answered yes. If you are older than 69 years of age and are not accustomed to being very active, you should always check with your doctor before changing your exercise routine.

Please read the following questions carefully and answer yes or no honestly to each one.

1. Has your doctor ever said that you have a heart condition and should only do physical activity recommended by a doctor?
2. Do you feel pain in your chest when you do physical activity?
3. In the past month, have you had chest pain when you were not engaged in physical activity?
4. Do you lose your balance because of dizziness, or do you ever lose consciousness?
5. Do you have a bone or joint problem (for example, back, knee, or hip) that could be made worse by a change in your physical activity?
6. Is your doctor currently prescribing drugs (for example, water pills) for blood pressure or a heart condition?
7. Do you know of any other reason why you should not do physical activity?

Please Note: If your health changes or you notice any of the above symptoms **after** you have already begun a fitness program, tell your fitness or health professional and ask whether you should change your physical activity plan.

Now, to help you make the most of your abilities, answer the following questions. Depending on your answers, you will take one of five different tracks.

Physical Fitness and Readiness Profile

1. **How often have you exercised in the last 4 weeks?**
   A. Not at all
   B. 1 to 4 times
   C. 5 to 8 times
   D. 9 to 12 times
   E. 13 or more times

2. **Right now, how many minutes nonstop can you perform weight-bearing cardio exercise, such as running or working on the elliptical trainer?**
   A. None
   B. Less than 12 minutes
   C. 13 to 30 minutes
   D. 31 to 59 minutes
   E. 60 to 75 minutes

3. **How many long push-ups can you perform without stopping? (Long push-ups are done with your legs straight and your knees off the ground. Short push-ups are done with both your knees and your toes on the ground.)**
   A. None
   B. 1 to 6 push-ups
   C. 7 to 12 push-ups
   D. 13 to 25 push-ups
   E. 26 to 100 push-ups

4. **Right now, how many full-range free squats can you perform in 60 seconds?**
   A. None
   B. 1 to 20
   C. 21 to 36
   D. 37 to 52
   E. 53 to 75

Scoring Key

A = 10
B = 8
C = 6
D = 4
E = 2

If you scored 33–40, you will take the **Red Track**.
If you scored 25–32, you will take the **Green Track**.
If you scored 17–24, you will take the **Orange Track**.
If you scored 9–16, you will take the **Yellow Track**.
If you scored 8, you will take the **Blue Track**.

GET MOVING

The following exercise programs are designed to help you get the most out of your workouts based on your own health and fitness level right now. As you become stronger, leaner, and fitter, you will be able to step up to the next level so that you continue to maximize your results.

Please note that wherever I refer to walking, running, or stationary biking, you can use any other appropriate exercise equipment, such as the elliptical trainer or treadmill, that is available to you.

Red Track

GOAL: Begin with 1 day a week and work your way up to 3 days a week performing 12 minutes of sustained activity. Once you can perform a total of three consecutive weeks of three exercise sessions a week consisting of at least 12 minutes of nonstop activity, move on to the **Green Track**.

MONDAY	WEDNESDAY	FRIDAY
12-minute walk	12-minute walk	12-minute walk
12-minute stationary bike	12-minute stationary bike	12-minute stationary bike
12-minute water aerobics	12-minute water aerobics	12-minute water aerobics

Green Track

GOAL: Exercise a minimum of 4 days a week. One of those days you will be performing one of my 12-minute CircuFit Workouts (see page 128). On the other days, perform 30 minutes of sustained activity, including 12 minutes of warmup and 6 minutes of cool down by walking or moving at a slower pace. Once you can perform a total of six rounds of my CircuFit Workout in the allotted 12 minutes, move on to the **Orange Track**.

MONDAY	TUESDAY	THURSDAY	FRIDAY
30-minute walk	12-minute CircuFit	30-minute walk	30-minute walk

Orange Track

GOAL: Exercise a minimum of 5 days a week. On two of those days you'll be doing one of my 12-minute CircuFit Workouts (see page 128). On the other days, perform 12 to 30 minutes of sustained activity whenever possible. Once you can perform a total of eight rounds of my CircuFit Workout in the allotted 12 minutes, move on to the **Yellow Track**.

MONDAY	TUESDAY	WEDNESDAY	THURSDAY	FRIDAY
30-minute walk	12-minute CircuFit	30-minute walk	12-minute CircuFit	30-minute walk

Yellow Track

GOAL: Exercise a minimum of 5 days a week, doing one of my 12-minute CircuFit Workouts (see page 128) on two of those days and running for 30 minutes on alternate days. Once you can perform a total of 10 rounds of my CircuFit Workout in the allotted 12 minutes, move on to the **Blue Track**.

MONDAY	TUESDAY	WEDNESDAY	THURSDAY	FRIDAY
30-minute run	12-minute CircuFit	30-minute run	12-minute CircuFit	30-minute run

Blue Track

GOAL: Exercise a minimum of 6 days a week, doing one of my 12-minute CircuFit Workouts (see page 128) on three of those days and doing 30 minutes of cardio activity or working out on your preferred cardio equipment on the alternate days. Once you can perform a total of 12 rounds of my CircuFit Workout in the allotted 12 minutes, keep track of your time and see if you can break your personal best record! If you complete 12 rounds in fewer than 12 minutes, your workout is over and you should start to cool down.

MONDAY	TUESDAY	WEDNESDAY	THURSDAY	FRIDAY	SATURDAY
12-minute CircuFit	30-minute run	12-minute CircuFit	30-minute elliptical	12-minute CircuFit	30-minute run

TWO 12-MINUTE CIRCUFIT PROGRAMS

The 12-minute CircuFit Workouts are exercise routines I created so that people could work out with minimal equipment in their homes, while traveling, outdoors if they prefer, and even at a health club. Ideally you will need a set of one-, two-, or five-pound dumbbells. Or continue using the weight you are accustomed to exercising with. If you don't have dumbbells, you can still perform the routines. Either use water bottles or cans of beans, or do the routines without the added weight until you are strong enough to add weight.

CircuFit is a form of circuit training that integrates multimuscle movements in a specific order so that the body is worked from head to toe. The workouts are designed to build muscle strength and endurance, cardiorespiratory health, balance, and flexibility, and to develop total body conditioning to maximize fat loss.

The two CircuFit Workout routines I have provided here are of equal difficulty and equally efficient. My goal is to give you some variety so that you are less likely to get bored. Once you have mastered the two routines provided here, visit my website (www.dietfreelife.com) for additional programs.

To perform a 12-minute CircuFit Workout, you need to warm up for 6 to 12 minutes and cool down for 5 to 10 minutes, which means that the total time of your workout will be about 30 minutes.

12 minutes warming up
+ 12 minutes CircuFit Workout
+　6 minutes cooling down
= 30 minutes

Baseline Boogie

WARM-UP: Slowly perform two sets of four repetitions of each of the three exercises, focusing on technique and range of motion. Going through the circuit twice in this manner is a great rehearsal and a muscle-specific warm-up. You can also begin warming up by marching in place before slowly performing the two warm-up sets (rounds) of the workout routine.

WORKOUT: Perform 12 repetitions of each exercise. Once you have performed all three exercises, you have completed a round. The goal is to perform as many rounds as possible with proper form and technique in 12 minutes.

▶ Free Squat and Overhead Shoulder Press

Standing with your feet shoulder-width apart, count to two as you slowly bend your knees, keeping your abdominals contracted and back straight, until your thighs are at a 90-degree angle. Straighten up, and once you are back at the starting position, keep your abdominals contracted and extend your arms up over your head with your palms facing each other. Then return to the starting position. This completes one repetition of this exercise. Continue until you have completed 12 repetitions.

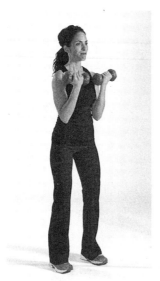

Starting position

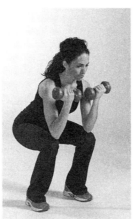

Descent of free squat

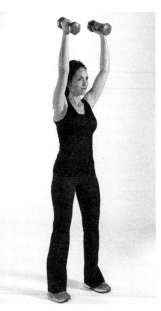

Overhead shoulder press to complete repetition

▶ Lateral Skater Leaps

Standing with your right leg off the ground and your arms extended straight out to the sides, hop over (or step over) to your right leg and touch your left hand to your right thigh, knee, shin, or the top of your foot. The lower you touch, the higher the intensity of the movement. Once you touch the targeted area, you have completed one repetition (second photo). Immediately hop over to the opposite leg and repeat with the opposite hand for a second repetition (third photo). Continue doing this until you've completed 12 repetitions.

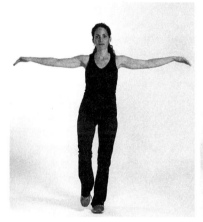

Starting position

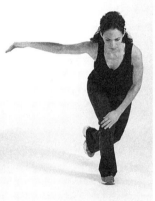

Leap over to opposite leg for one repetition

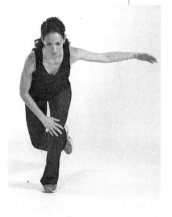

Leap back to the opposite leg for a second repetition, and so on

▶ Push-Ups

Lying face down, place your hands on the floor slightly below your shoulders and just wider than shoulder-width apart. Raise your hips so that they are level with your trunk, and bend your knees so that your body weight is evenly distributed. You have the option of performing a short or long push-up. The difference is that when performing a short push-up, both your knees and toes are on the ground; when performing a long push-up, your legs are straight and only your toes and hands are on the ground. Also, if you aren't able to exercise on the ground, you can stand and do a wall push-up.

During the active phase of the exercise, slowly lower your body to the floor—stopping when your elbows are level with your trunk (at a 90-degree angle). Exhale as you push up to the starting position, keeping your elbows slightly bent. Continue until you have completed 12 repetitions.

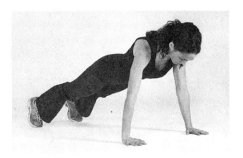

Starting position

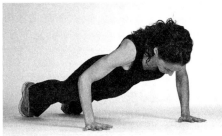

Descend until arms are at right angles

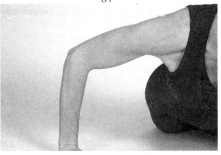

The angle to which you want to descend when performing a push-up

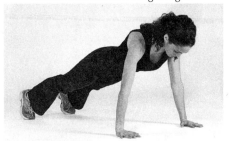

Return to starting position to complete repetition

COOL DOWN: Take 6 minutes to cool down. Walk in place or go for a slow walk outside or on a treadmill. The most important thing is to continue moving and drinking water as your body cools down.

Super Set Slim Down

WARM-UP: Slowly perform two sets of four repetitions of each of the three exercises, focusing on technique and range of motion. Going through the circuit twice in this manner is a great rehearsal and a muscle-specific warm-up. You can also begin warming up by marching in place before slowly performing the two warm-up sets (rounds) of the workout routine.

WORKOUT: Perform 12 repetitions of each exercise. Once you have performed all three exercises, you have completed a round. The goal is to perform as many rounds as possible with proper form and technique in 12 minutes.

▶ Alternating Lunges with Overhead Shoulder Press

Standing with your feet shoulder-width apart, step backward while keeping your feet the same distance apart, toes pointing straight ahead. Elevate your back heel to transfer your weight to the front heel and mid-foot. While keeping your back straight, chest lifted, and abs contracted, lower your back knee until it is at a 45-degree angle to the floor (see second photo), then advance to a 90-degree angle, as shown in the third photo. Exhale as you return to the starting position, keeping your knees slightly bent. Then, perform an overhead shoulder press, with your palms facing each other. Return to the starting position. Step back with the other leg and repeat. Continue for 12 repetitions, with every overhead shoulder press making for one repetition.

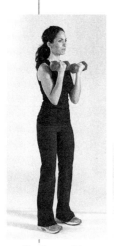

Starting position

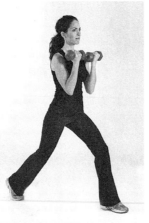

Step back and establish balance

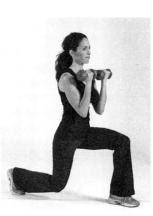

Descent of stationary lunge

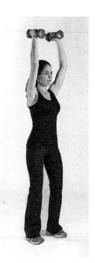

Return to starting position and perform overhead shoulder press to complete repetition

Diet-Free for Life

▶ Straddle Split

Start by standing with your feet together, then simultaneously position both feet about 2 feet apart with your toes pointing slightly outward. With your weight on your heels, lower your hips while keeping your back straight. Reach down with both hands and touch your knees, your shins, or the tops of your feet, then return to the starting position with your feet together for one repetition. Continue for 12 repetitions.

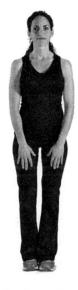

Starting position

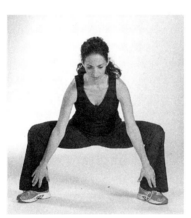

Turn outward and perform a squat, like a ballet plié

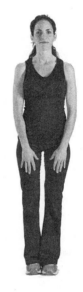

Return to starting position to complete repetition

▶ Standing Chest Fly

Stand with your feet shoulder-width apart and your arms out to the sides at a 90-degree angle. Your elbows should be at shoulder height, and your palms should be facing forward. Keeping your back straight, abdominals contracted, and knees slightly bent, slowly move your elbows, forearms, and palms toward each other, as if closing a door. Once your arms are a few inches from touching, contract your chest muscles while exhaling. Then return to the starting position for the completion of one repetition. Continue for a total of 12 repetitions.

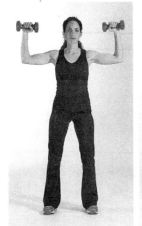 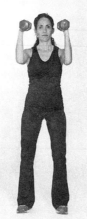 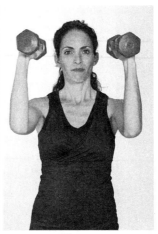 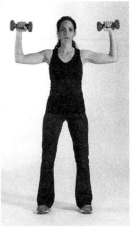

Starting position   *Bring arms forward and contract chest muscles*   *Close up*   *Return to starting position to complete repetition*

COOL DOWN: Take 6 minutes to cool down. Walk in place or go for a slow walk outside or on a treadmill. The most important thing is to continue moving and drinking water as your body cools down.

11

Fat Loss Recipes

MAIN DISHES

Some of these recipes will make a complete fat-burning meal on their own, and others can be paired with your favorite sides.

Chicken O'Delicious

MAKES 4 SERVINGS

This Mexican-flavored chicken dish looks complicated, but it's really easy to make. (I recommend serving with ½ to ⅔ cup black beans for women, ⅔ to ¾ cup for men.)

- 4 (4-ounce) skinless and boneless chicken breasts
- 2 tablespoons extra-virgin olive oil
- 2 tablespoons balsamic vinegar
- ⅓ cup sun-dried tomatoes, packed in oil
- 1 tablespoon minced garlic
- 1 (16-ounce) jar prepared salsa verde
- 1 (15-ounce) can black beans, drained

Cut the chicken into bite-size pieces. In a large saucepan over medium heat, combine the oil and vinegar. Add the tomatoes and garlic, and sauté until tender. Add the chicken and cook on medium heat until chicken is not pink in the middle. Add the salsa and black beans, and simmer 5 minutes.

Per serving: 379.3 calories, 42.3 grams protein, 30.8 grams carbohydrates, 11.6 grams fat, 6.3 grams fiber

MAIN DISHES

Serve this Indian-inspired chicken with a side dish of cucumber salad or another salad of your choice.

2¼ cups plain nonfat Greek yogurt

2½ tablespoons freshly squeezed lemon juice

1½ tablespoons extra-virgin olive oil

1 teaspoon freshly ground black pepper

1 teaspoon chili powder

1 teaspoon ground cumin

6 (4-ounce) skinless and boneless chicken breasts

½ cup finely chopped fresh mint leaves

3 tablespoons diced green onion

¾ cup whole fresh mint leaves

In a small bowl, combine 1 cup of the yogurt, 1 tablespoon of the lemon juice, and 1 tablespoon of the oil; then mix in the black pepper, chili powder, and cumin. Add the chicken and turn until well coated. Marinate at room temperature for about 20 to 30 minutes.

Stir together the remaining 1¼ cups of yogurt, the remaining 1½ tablespoons of lemon juice, and the chopped mint leaves. Set aside.

Spray a grill pan with nonstick cooking spray and set it over medium heat. When the pan is hot, discard the marinade and grill the chicken over indirect heat, turning occasionally, until the juices run clear, 18 to 20 minutes. Watch carefully to prevent burning.

Transfer the chicken to a serving platter.

In a small bowl, toss together the remaining ½ tablespoon of the oil, the green onion, and the whole mint leaves. Drizzle the chicken with the yogurt sauce, and top with the green onion and mint mixture.

Per serving: 266.2 calories, 43.6 grams protein, 4.5 grams carbohydrates, 7.7 grams fat, 0.6 grams fiber

MAIN DISHES

Sweet Grilled Chicken

Serve this honey-glazed chicken with a side of spinach salad and brown rice in the amount of ½ cup for women, ⅔ cup for men.

½ cup honey (organic if possible)

2 tablespoons freshly squeezed lemon juice

¼ teaspoon curry powder

1 clove garlic, crushed

1 tablespoon mustard seeds

1 tablespoon Dijon mustard

3 tablespoons light butter

1 tablespoon minced green onion

6 (4-ounce) skinless and boneless chicken breasts

½ teaspoon freshly ground black pepper

Combine the honey, lemon juice, curry powder, garlic, and mustard seeds in a small saucepan over medium heat, stirring frequently until hot and well blended. Whisk in the mustard, butter, and green onion, and keep warm.

Lightly coat a grill pan with nonstick cooking spray and set it over medium-high heat. Season the chicken with the black pepper and grill, basting frequently with the warm sauce. Cook 15 to 20 minutes, turning occasionally.

Transfer the chicken to a serving platter and drizzle with the remaining sauce.

Per serving: 235.7 calories, 35.7 grams protein, 4.8 grams carbohydrates, 7.1 grams fat, 0.4 grams fiber

MAIN DISHES

The sweetness of honey is the perfect foil for the tangy lemon in this grilled chicken recipe.

MAKES 6 SERVINGS

- 2–3 tablespoons freshly squeezed lemon juice
- 1 tablespoon distilled white vinegar
- 2 tablespoons chopped fresh dill
- 2 tablespoons chopped fresh basil
- 1 tablespoon honey (organic if possible)
- 1 tablespoon honey Dijon mustard
- ¼ teaspoon freshly ground black pepper
- ¼ cup extra-virgin olive oil
- 6 (4-ounce) skinless and boneless chicken breasts, lightly pounded
- 1 lemon, thinly sliced
- ⅓ cup pitted kalamata olives, halved

Preheat the grill to medium-high heat.

To make the dressing, whisk together the lemon juice, vinegar, dill, basil, honey, mustard, and black pepper. Slowly whisk in the oil.

Place the chicken in a large sealable plastic bag. Add half the lemon slices and ⅓ cup of the dressing. Close the bag and refrigerate for at least 2 hours, turning at least once. Add the rest of the lemon slices and the olives to the remaining dressing.

When ready to cook, discard the marinade and grill the chicken until it is no longer pink in the middle, 5 to 6 minutes per side.

Serve with the honey-lemon dressing.

Per serving: 274 calories, 26.3 grams protein, 5.9 grams carbohydrates, 15.6 grams fat, 0.4 grams fiber

MAIN DISHES

Stuffed and Puffed Chicken Breasts

**MAKES 4
SERVINGS**

Enjoy these delectable stuffed chicken breasts with one of your favorite fast carbs to create a perfect fat-burning meal.

4 (4-ounce) skinless and boneless chicken breasts

2 tablespoons extra-virgin olive oil

1 teaspoon dried thyme

¼ teaspoon crushed red pepper flakes

1 (7-ounce) jar artichoke hearts, drained, rinsed, and chopped

2 teaspoons minced garlic

¼ teaspoon freshly ground black pepper

3 ounces herbed goat cheese, crumbled

3 tablespoons drained and minced sun-dried tomatoes, packed in oil

2 tablespoons finely chopped fresh basil

Additional garlic and freshly ground black pepper, for finishing

Preheat the grill to medium heat.

Rinse the chicken breasts under cold water and pat them dry. Place each breast between 2 sheets of plastic wrap and gently beat with mallet to flatten to ¼ inch thick.

Warm 1 tablespoon of the oil with the thyme and red pepper flakes in a medium sauté pan over medium-high heat for 1 to 2 minutes. Add the artichoke hearts, garlic, and black pepper, and cook for 3 to 4 minutes, stirring occasionally.

Remove the pan from the heat; add the goat cheese, tomatoes, and basil, and mix to distribute the ingredients evenly. Set the stuffing aside to cool.

Spread each breast half with a quarter of the cooled stuffing. Fold the breasts in half over the stuffing and use toothpicks to hold them closed.

Brush both sides of each breast with the remaining tablespoon of oil, and season with additional garlic and black pepper. Grill over medium heat, turning once, until the meat juices run clear and the cheese is melted, 8 to 12 minutes. Remove from the grill and carefully remove the toothpicks.

Per serving: 332.8 calories, 40.6 grams protein, 2.6 grams carbohydrates, 15.6 grams fat, 1.4 grams fiber

MAIN DISHES

Broiled chicken with black bean sauce and a variety of vegetables makes a wonderful meal for you and your family or friends. Just add ½ cup brown rice or any other slow carb to make a perfect fat-burning meal.

3 tablespoons diced yellow onion

½ teaspoon minced garlic

1 cup chicken stock

1 (14-ounce) can black beans, rinsed and drained

¼ cup diced tomatoes

½ teaspoon minced fresh cilantro

2 teaspoons ground dried chipotle chilies

1 tablespoon extra-virgin olive oil

2 tablespoons chili powder

4 (4-ounce) skinless and boneless chicken breasts

Lightly spray a large saucepan with nonstick cooking spray. Sauté the onions and garlic over medium heat until the onions are translucent. Add the chicken stock, beans, tomatoes, cilantro, and chilies, and simmer until slightly thickened, 15 to 20 minutes. Remove from the heat and set aside to cool. Puree half the bean mixture in a blender or food processor, transfer to a bowl, add the rest of the bean mixture, and mix well.

Preheat the broiler.

Combine the oil and chili powder in a small bowl to make a paste. Brush the paste over the chicken breasts.

Broil the chicken 3 to 5 minutes per side, or until cooked through. Top with the black bean sauce and serve.

Per serving: 256 calories, 32.9 grams protein, 6.2 grams carbohydrates, 4.9 grams fat, 5.4 grams fiber

MAIN DISHES

Easy Lemon-Crusted Chicken

MAKES 4 SERVINGS

Enjoy the taste of Italy right in your own kitchen. Just add some steamed veggies or a colorful salad, and you have a complete fat-burning meal.

⅔ cup whole wheat bread crumbs

½ cup freshly grated Parmesan cheese (or rice or soy cheese)

¼ teaspoon dried oregano

¼ cup dried parsley

4 tablespoons freshly ground black pepper

4 tablespoons minced lemon zest

4 (4-ounce) skinless and boneless chicken breasts

Preheat the oven to 450°F. Coat a baking pan with nonstick cooking spray.

In a mixing bowl, combine the bread crumbs, cheese, oregano, parsley, and black pepper.

Coat both sides of the chicken breasts with the bread crumb mixture and place in the prepared pan. Sprinkle each breast with 1 tablespoon lemon zest and bake for 22 to 28 minutes, or until lightly browned and cooked through.

Per serving: 206 calories, 30 grams protein, 11.6 grams carbohydrates, 5.5 grams fat, 1.9 grams fiber

MAIN DISHES

Sweet and Spicy Korean Chicken

When you're in the mood for something with a kick, this Korean spiced dish is the way to go. Serve it with ½ cup brown rice or two low-carb whole wheat tortillas for a complete fat-burning meal.

MAKES 2 SERVINGS

2 tablespoons extra-virgin olive oil

½ apple, cut into chunks

1 celery stalk, cut into chunks

½ green bell pepper, cored, seeded, and cut into chunks

⅓ medium onion, cut into bite-size pieces

¾ pound skinless and boneless chicken tenderloins, cut into chunks

1 tablespoon gochujang (Korean hot pepper paste)

¼ cup dry white wine

Pinch lemon pepper

2 tablespoons evaporated cane juice*

1 tablespoon minced garlic

Pinch freshly ground black pepper

Heat the oil in a large skillet over medium heat. Stir in the apple, celery, bell pepper, and onion, and cook until the onion is softened and translucent, about 5 minutes.

Stir in the chicken, gochujang, wine, lemon pepper, cane juice, garlic, and black pepper. Cook until the chicken is no longer pink in the center, about 5 minutes.

Per serving: 430.5 calories, 48 grams protein, 18.6 grams carbohydrates, 17.7 grams fat, 2.3 grams fiber

*In place of evaporated cane juice, you can use natural brown sugar, granulated Splenda, or raw sugar, just to name a few. For additional ingredient alternatives, go to www.dietfreelife.com.

MAIN DISHES

**MAKES 4
SERVINGS**

This blend of Southwest favorites makes an ideal fat-burning meal for four.

For the dressing

¼ cup low-fat sour cream

1 cup plain nonfat Greek yogurt

2 tablespoons freshly squeezed lime juice

1 teaspoon grated lime zest

1 teaspoon hot paprika

¼ teaspoon freshly ground black pepper

¼ teaspoon cayenne pepper

8 drops hot pepper sauce

For the fajitas

1 teaspoon extra-virgin olive oil

4 (4-ounce) skinless and boneless chicken breasts, cut into 1-inch pieces

¼ teaspoon freshly ground black pepper

1 medium red onion, chopped into ½-inch pieces

12 cherry tomatoes, halved

4 cups fresh salad greens

4 large low-carb whole wheat tortillas, warmed

Make the dressing: In a medium bowl, combine all the dressing ingredients. Refrigerate for at least 30 minutes or until ready to serve.

Make the fajitas: Pour the oil into a large nonstick skillet over medium-high heat. Add the chicken and pepper, and cook for 3 minutes. Turn the chicken pieces and cook for 3 to 4 more minutes. Add the onion and tomatoes, and mix well. Continue to cook until the chicken is golden brown on the outside and no longer pink on the inside, and the juices are beginning to caramelize on the skillet's edge. Remove from the heat.

Place 1 cup salad greens on each tortilla and top with one-quarter of the chicken. Drizzle 2 to 3 tablespoons of dressing over each serving.

Per serving: 478.5 calories, 67.9 grams protein, 37.9 grams carbohydrates, 12.3 grams fat, 14.8 grams fiber

MAIN DISHES

Grilled to Perfection Chicken Burritos

Packed with grilled vegetables, chicken, and cheese, and topped with your favorite salsa, these tasty burritos make an extraordinary fat-burning meal.

4 (4-ounce) skinless and boneless chicken breasts

½ red bell pepper, cored, seeded, and cut into ½-inch-wide strips

½ green bell pepper, cored, seeded, and cut into ½-inch-wide strips

1 small onion, sliced into thin slivers

¼ cup extra-virgin olive oil

2 tablespoons freshly squeezed lime juice

2 cloves garlic, minced

1 teaspoon chili powder

4 large low-carb, low-fat tortillas

1 cup shredded Monterey Jack cheese (or rice or soy cheese)

8 tablespoons salsa of your choice

Place the chicken in an 11 × 7 inch glass baking dish; scatter the bell peppers and onion slices over the chicken. In a small jar, combine 3 tablespoons of the oil with the lime juice, garlic, and chili powder. Cover tightly and shake to blend. Pour the mixture over the chicken and vegetables, cover, and refrigerate for 1 to 2 hours.

Preheat the grill to medium-high.

Place a 12 by 18-inch sheet of heavy-duty foil on a work surface. Remove the peppers and onions from the chicken, letting the marinade drip back into the baking dish, and place them on the foil.

Wrap the vegetables in the foil and grill for 10 minutes, turning once. Move the packet to the side. Drain the chicken, place it on the grill, and cook, covered, for 6 to 7 minutes per side, or until the juices run clear.

Remove the chicken and vegetables but don't turn off the grill.

Slice the chicken into thin strips. Place a quarter of the strips in a line down the center of a tortilla. Add a quarter of the vegetables and ¼ cup of the cheese. Don't overfill the tortilla. Fold the short ends of the tortilla over the filling, then fold over the long sides and roll up tightly. Repeat with the remaining tortillas and filling.

MAIN DISHES

Brush the remaining 1 tablespoon of oil over the burritos and grill, seam side down, until firm and browned, about 2 minutes. Turn and grill for 2 more minutes. Serve topped with 2 tablespoons of salsa.

Per serving: 550.5 calories, 49.5 grams protein, 26.3 grams carbohydrates, 35.5 grams fat, 15.1 grams fiber

This garlicky hot chicken panini makes a zingy fat-burning sandwich.

**MAKES 4
SERVINGS**

4 (4-ounce) skinless and boneless chicken breasts

2 tablespoons chopped garlic

1 tablespoon freshly ground black pepper

2 medium red bell peppers

1 tablespoon extra-virgin olive oil

8 slices sourdough bread

¼ cup honey mustard

8 (½-ounce) slices provolone cheese (or rice or soy cheese)

12 basil leaves

¼ pound pepperoni

½ cup grated mozzarella cheese (or rice or soy cheese)

Preheat the grill to medium.

Sprinkle the chicken breasts with the garlic and black pepper, and grill until browned and cooked through, 7 minutes on each side. Place the chicken on a cutting board, cool, and then cut into strips and set aside.

Brush the red peppers lightly with the oil, and grill until the skin is charred and black all over, about 20 minutes. Put the grilled peppers in a paper bag, close the bag, and wait about 5 minutes. Remove the peppers from the bag and rub off the charred skin. Remove the seeds and stems, and cut the peppers into strips.

Place sourdough slices on the grill until toasted to your preferred doneness on one side. Transfer to a plate, toasted side down, and spread 4 of the slices with 1 tablespoon of the mustard. Top with 2 slices of the provolone; 3 basil leaves; 1 ounce of pepperoni; and one-quarter each of the chicken, red peppers, and mozzarella. Top with the other slice of bread, toasted side up.

Wrap the sandwiches in aluminum foil, reduce the heat on the grill to low, and grill the sandwiches, turning once, for 7 minutes, or until cheese is melted. Remove from foil, slice each sandwich in half, and serve.

Per serving: 515 calories, 55.4 grams protein, 34 grams carbohydrates, 17 grams fat, 7.2 grams fiber

MAIN DISHES

MAKES 2 SERVINGS

Fresh apricots and tarragon combined with grilled chicken make this salad the essence of summer and a complete fat-burning meal.

3 (4-ounce) skinless and boneless chicken breasts, pounded to ½-inch thick

1 tablespoon minced fresh flat-leaf parsley

2 teaspoons minced fresh tarragon

¼ teaspoon freshly ground black pepper

3 tablespoons extra-virgin olive oil

4 teaspoons white wine vinegar

4 cups baby arugula leaves

4 cups mesclun or other baby salad greens

3 apricots (8 ounces total), pitted and thinly sliced

⅓ cup thinly sliced red onion

Preheat the grill to medium-high. Spray the grill rack with nonstick cooking spray.

Sprinkle the chicken breast with the parsley, tarragon, and black pepper.

Grill the breasts until cooked through, 4 minutes on each side. Transfer to a plate and set aside to cool.

In a small bowl, whisk together the oil, vinegar, and a dash of black pepper.

Place the arugula, mesclun, apricots, and onion in a large bowl, and toss with the dressing. Divide the salad between 2 plates. Cut the chicken breast into thin slices and arrange them on top of the greens. Serve immediately.

Per serving: 425.6 calories, 27.4 grams protein, 24.8 grams carbohydrates, 22.8 grams fat, 7.4 grams fiber

MAIN DISHES

Chicken Mango Splash Salad

This quick and easy salad uses just the right combination of chicken, fresh greens, ripe mangos, and sliced almonds to create a dynamic lunch to be served with a fast carb such as rice or couscous.

MAKES 4 SERVINGS

1 (10-ounce) can white meat chicken, drained

1 mango, peeled, pitted, and cut into ¼-inch cubes (1 cup)

1 celery stalk, minced (½ cup)

¼ cup minced fresh flat-leaf parsley

1 cup plain nonfat Greek yogurt

1 tablespoon freshly squeezed lemon juice

¼ teaspoon freshly ground black pepper

4 cups fresh salad greens

¼ cup sliced almonds

Combine the chicken, mango, celery, parsley, yogurt, lemon juice, and black pepper in a medium bowl.

Divide the salad greens among 4 plates and scoop about ¾ cup chicken-mango mixture on top of each plate.

Top each serving with 1 teaspoon of sliced almonds.

Per serving: 177 calories, 23.4 grams protein, 12.5 grams carbohydrates, 3.7 grams fat, 6.7 grams fiber

MAIN DISHES

Served with steamed vegetables, this slow-cooked casserole makes an ideal fat-burning meal that's certainly worth the wait. If you don't have a slow cooker, don't stress; just cook it slowly in a heavy casserole on top of the stove.

4 ounces long-grain wild rice

14 ounces low-sodium chicken broth

1 can low-fat cream of chicken soup

1 cup skim milk

4 (4-ounce) skinless and boneless chicken breasts, sliced

1 cup sliced water chestnuts

⅔ cup plain protein powder

Hot paprika, for garnish

Put the rice in a slow cooker. In a medium bowl, whisk together the chicken broth, cream of chicken soup, and milk. Pour half the mixture over the rice and stir.

Add the chicken breasts and water chestnuts to the slow cooker, and then add the remaining soup mixture.

Cover and cook on low for 4 to 6 hours, or until the rice is tender and the chicken is cooked through.

Just before serving, whisk the protein powder into the chicken and rice mixture to thicken the sauce. Sprinkle with paprika and serve.

Per serving: 405 calories, 55.5 grams protein, 27.5 grams carbohydrates, 7.5 grams fat, 1.8 grams fiber

MAIN DISHES

This comfort soup goes well with a biscuit or with ½ cup rice for women, ⅔ cup for men.

1 cup canned corn, drained

3¾ cups chicken broth

12 ounces cooked chicken breast, cut into strips

16 baby corn cobs

1 teaspoon Chinese curry powder

1 (½-inch) piece fresh gingerroot, grated

3 tablespoons low-sodium soy sauce

2 tablespoons diced fresh chives

Place the canned corn in a food processor with ⅔ cup of the broth and puree until smooth.

Strain the corn puree through a fine sieve, pressing gently with the back of a spoon to separate the coverings of the kernels.

In a large pot, combine the remaining broth, the chicken strips, and the corn puree. Mix well.

Add the baby corn cobs and bring the mixture to a boil. Reduce the heat to medium and cook for 10 minutes.

Add the curry powder, ginger, and soy sauce, and stir well. Cook for another 10 to 15 minutes.

Stir in the chives, pour into four bowls, and serve.

Per serving: 154.62 calories, 23 grams protein, 13.16 grams carbohydrates, 1.59 grams fat, 3 grams fiber

MAIN DISHES

Chicken Taco Soup

The warmth of this Mexican-style main course soup will keep you in toasty fat-burning mode no matter how cold it is outside.

½ cup diced onion

½ cup diced green bell pepper

1 tablespoon minced garlic

½ tablespoon extra-virgin olive oil

4 (4-ounce) skinless and boneless chicken breasts, boiled and shredded

1 (1.25-ounce) package taco seasoning mix

1 (8-ounce) jar salsa

1 (7-ounce) can corn kernels, drained

1 (14-ounce) can hominy, drained

1 (16-ounce) can ranch-style beans, drained

2 (4-ounce) cans tomato paste

2 (14-ounce) cans low-sodium chicken broth

1 (8-ounce) package light cream cheese

In a large stockpot, sauté the onion, bell pepper, and garlic in the oil. Add the chicken, taco seasoning, salsa, corn, hominy, beans, tomato paste, and chicken broth. Bring to a slow simmer and simmer for 20 minutes.

Place the cream cheese in a bowl, remove some of the hot liquid from the soup, and pour it over the cream cheese. Stir to melt the cheese, and then pour the mixture back into the stockpot.

Simmer on low for another 10 minutes.

Serve with a few tortilla chips and ¼ cup grated Cheddar cheese for women, ⅓ cup Cheddar cheese for men. Be sure to keep a close eye on the serving size of the chips.

Per serving (without chips and grated cheese): 321.6 calories, 31.7 grams protein, 39.6 grams carbohydrates, 4.3 grams fat, 9.8 grams fiber

MAIN DISHES

Diet-Free for Life

Personalize these spicy turkey patties with your own favorite toppings and condiments.

MAKES 4 SERVINGS

For the sauce

½ cup ketchup

1 tablespoon balsamic vinegar

1 tablespoon Worcestershire sauce

2 cloves garlic, minced

¼ teaspoon crushed red pepper flakes

¼ teaspoon hot sauce

¼ teaspoon freshly ground black pepper

For the burgers

1 pound ground turkey

⅓ cup quick-cooking oats

Preheat the grill to medium-high.

Make the sauce: In a small bowl, combine all the sauce ingredients and set aside.

Make the burgers: Combine the turkey and oats in a large bowl. Add half the sauce and mix thoroughly. Form into 4 equal patties.

Grill for 5 to 7 minutes per side, basting with the remaining sauce after burgers have been turned.

Per serving: 171.8 calories, 35.3 grams protein, 7 grams carbohydrates, 1.8 grams fat, 0.7 grams fiber

MAIN DISHES

The tomato and basil pasta sauce gives these burgers a true Italian taste.

1 pound ground turkey

½ cup prepared tomato and basil pasta sauce

⅓ cup finely chopped onion

¼ cup whole wheat bread crumbs

¼ cup freshly grated Parmesan cheese (or rice or soy cheese)

1 tablespoon dried parsley

¼ teaspoon minced garlic

4 (1-ounce) slices fat-free mozzarella cheese (or rice or soy cheese)

2 whole wheat pitas split in half horizontally

1 clove garlic, halved

Lettuce and tomato for serving (optional)

In mixing bowl, combine the turkey, pasta sauce, onion, bread crumbs, Parmesan cheese, parsley, and minced garlic, mixing it gently with your hands. Divide into 4 equal patties.

Heat a grill pan over medium heat and grill the burgers until cooked through, 6 to 7 minutes per side. Top each with a mozzarella cheese slice and cover the pan to melt the cheese. Rub the inside of each pita half with the cut garlic and toast them in the toaster oven. Place a burger on each half pita, and serve with lettuce and tomato, if using.

Per serving: 470.3 calories, 46.6 grams protein, 31.9 grams carbohydrates, 18.1 grams fat, 6.3 grams fiber

MAIN DISHES

MAKES 1 SERVING

The creaminess of avocado pairs with hummus and cucumber for a taste that's out of this world. This quick and easy recipe makes a complete fat-burning meal in less than 15 minutes. Vegetarians can replace the turkey with a meat substitute.

2 corn tortillas

¼ cup prepared hummus

½ avocado, sliced thinly

¼ cucumber, sliced

¼ cup baby spinach leaves

2 slices nitrate-free deli turkey

Warm the tortillas in the microwave for 1 minute. Divide the remaining ingredients equally between the tortillas, roll up, and serve.

Per serving: 385 calories, 17.6 grams protein, 42.7 grams carbohydrates, 19.2 grams fat, 11.5 grams fiber

MAIN DISHES

Chipotle Turkey Wrap

These tangy turkey wraps make a tasty fat-burning meal for the entire family.

For the chipotle sauce

1 tablespoon light cream cheese, softened

2 tablespoons light butter

2 tablespoons light sour cream

1 teaspoon red wine vinegar

1 chipotle pepper in adobo sauce, seeded and finely chopped

For the wraps

2 ears fresh corn, husked

2 tablespoons light butter

2 tablespoons chopped fresh garlic

1 teaspoon freshly ground black pepper

1 teaspoon chopped flat-leaf parsley

1 teaspoon chopped fresh cilantro

2 tablespoons chopped red bell pepper

2 tablespoons chopped red onion

1 tablespoon red wine vinegar

2 tablespoons freshly squeezed lime juice

6 whole wheat tortilla wraps

¼ pound light pepper Jack cheese, cut into 6 slices

¼ pound Muenster cheese, cut into 6 slices

6 red leaf lettuce leaves

1 avocado, thinly sliced

1 pound cooked turkey breast, thinly sliced

Make the chipotle sauce: Combine all the ingredients in a small mixing bowl, cover, and refrigerate for at least ½ hour.

Preheat the grill to high.

Make the wraps: Place corn on a large piece of heavy-duty foil, top with the butter, garlic, and black pepper. Make a foil packet by wrapping the corn tightly, and grill for 20 minutes, turning it once or twice. Unwrap and set aside to cool.

MAIN DISHES

Diet-Free for Life

When the corn is cool enough to handle, cut the kernels from the cobs and put them in a mixing bowl. Mix in the parsley, cilantro, bell pepper, onion, vinegar, and lime juice. Refrigerate for at least ½ hour.

Lay a tortilla wrap on a work surface and layer with 1 slice each of the pepper Jack and Muenster cheese, 1 lettuce leaf, and one-sixth of the avocado and reserved corn relish. Drizzle with some of the chipotle sauce, and top with one-sixth of the turkey. Roll up to form a wrap. Repeat with the remaining ingredients.

Per serving: 391.2 calories, 35.4 grams protein, 38.9 grams carbohydrates, 16.3 grams fat, 15.5 grams fiber

**MAKES 8
SERVINGS**

Fresh turkey breast rolled around tender vegetables and accompanied by steamed broccoli and warm couscous makes a delightful fat-burning meal.

8 (5-ounce) pieces of skinless and boneless turkey breast

Freshly ground black pepper

¾ cup diced onion

½ cup thinly sliced celery

½ cup coarsely chopped carrot

1 tablespoon light butter

½ cup whole wheat bread crumbs

2 tablespoons white wine or water

1 teaspoon mixed dried herbs of your choice

½ cup low-sodium chicken broth

1 tablespoon extra-virgin olive oil

Preheat the grill to high. Soak 6 (18-inch) lengths of heavy-duty kitchen string in water.

Butterfly each piece of turkey breast by slicing almost but not quite all the way through horizontally and opening it up like a book. Cover with plastic wrap and pound to even the surface, no more than 1 inch thick. Remove the plastic and season the breasts with black pepper. Place the turkey pieces on a flat work surface.

In medium skillet over medium heat, sauté the onion, celery, and carrot in the butter until tender, about 7 minutes.

Remove from the heat and stir in the bread crumbs, wine, and mixed herbs.

Spread the vegetable mixture over the turkey, leaving a border all around.

Starting with the shorter edge, roll up each turkey piece, tucking in the edges as tightly as possible. Using the soaked string, tie each roll at 1-inch intervals.

Combine the chicken broth and oil in a measuring cup. Set a baking dish under the grill rack to catch the liquid. Put the turkey rolls on the rack and brush them with the broth mixture. With the lid down, grill for about 1 hour,

MAIN DISHES

or until the center reaches 170°F, brushing with the broth mixture every 15 minutes and rotating once or twice.

Remove from the grill, cover with foil, and let cool for 10 minutes before slicing.

Per serving: 238.1 calories, 43.6 grams protein, 5.5 grams carbohydrates, 3.4 grams fat, 1.7 grams fiber

**MAKES 9
SERVINGS**

You don't have to save this for a meal; try it as a snack as well.

3 ounces undiluted orange juice concentrate

3 cloves garlic, minced

¼ teaspoon hot paprika

1 tablespoon no-sugar-added orange marmalade

½ teaspoon low-sodium soy sauce

1 (3-pound) fresh or frozen and thawed turkey breast

2 teaspoons arrowroot or cornstarch mixed with 2 tablespoons cold water

Preheat oven to 350°F.

In a small bowl, combine orange juice concentrate, garlic, paprika, marmalade, and soy sauce.

Tear off a piece of heavy-duty aluminum foil long enough to completely wrap the entire turkey breast.

Place the turkey in the center of the foil and cover it on all sides with the orange mixture.

Wrap the turkey very tightly in the foil, being careful not to tear the foil. The point is to keep all the glaze inside while the turkey cooks. You can wrap the whole thing in a second piece of foil if necessary.

Place the foil-wrapped turkey in a shallow baking dish and bake in preheated oven for 3 hours. (Note: Do not open the foil to peek until the time is up.)

Remove the turkey from the oven, open the foil carefully, and drain the juices into a saucepan. Stir in the arrowroot mixture, and set over medium heat until thick and bubbly. Stir occasionally and keep covered.

Slice the turkey breast and serve with the orange glaze.

Per serving: 199 calories, 41 grams protein, 3 grams carbohydrates, 3.6 grams fat, 1.1 grams fiber

MAIN DISHES

Give your turkey a makeover with this Thai-inspired recipe. Serve it over ½ cup rice for women, ⅔ cup for men, to complete your fat-burning meal.

MAKES 4 SERVINGS

- 1 pound turkey breast
- 2 tablespoons extra-virgin olive oil
- 1 large onion, halved lengthwise and sliced thin
- ½ medium red bell pepper, cored, seeded, and cut into ½-inch strips, then halved crosswise
- 2 jalapeño peppers, seeded and minced
- ⅓ cup reduced-sodium chicken broth
- 3 large cloves garlic, minced
- 2 tablespoons low-sodium soy sauce
- 1 cup fresh mint leaves, chopped

Cut the turkey into 3 × ¼ × ½ inch strips and set aside. Heat 1 tablespoon of the oil over medium-high heat in a large skillet or wok. Add the onion, bell pepper, and jalapeño peppers, and sauté, stirring, for 3 minutes. Add 2 tablespoons of the broth, cover, and cook over medium heat until the onion browns slightly, about 3 minutes; it may still be a bit crunchy. Transfer the vegetable mixture to a bowl.

Add the remaining 1 tablespoon oil to the skillet and heat over medium-high heat. Add the turkey and sauté for 1 minute. Return the vegetable mixture to the skillet. Add the garlic, soy sauce, and remaining broth, and bring to a boil. Cover and cook over low heat for 2 minutes, or until the turkey is no longer pink inside. Add the mint and cook ½ minute.

Per serving: 237 calories, 34.8 grams protein, 4.8 grams carbohydrates, 8.3 grams fat, 1.1 grams fiber

MAIN DISHES

MAKES 4 SERVINGS

This loaded-with-vitamins soup has just the right balance of delicious turkey, fresh asparagus, and rich potatoes to create the perfect fat-burning meal for four.

4 (4-ounce) skinless turkey breast cutlets

8 small red potatoes, halved

4 cups water

1 teaspoon extra-virgin olive oil

1 small onion, cut into 1-inch pieces (½ cup)

1 pound asparagus, cut into 1-inch pieces (2 cups)

½ teaspoon freshly ground black pepper

2 cups low-fat milk or soymilk

¼ cup all-purpose unbleached flour

Place the turkey, potatoes, and water in a large saucepan, and bring to a boil. Cook over medium-high heat for about 7 minutes, or until the cutlets are no longer pink. Remove the turkey and cool to room temperature, then simmer the potatoes over low heat.

Meanwhile, put the oil in a skillet over medium heat and sauté the onion for 2 minutes. Add the asparagus and black pepper, and sauté for 2 more minutes. Add the onion and asparagus to the potatoes, and cook until the asparagus is tender but not limp, 5 to 7 minutes. Dice the turkey into ¼-inch pieces and add them to the saucepan, adjusting the heat so that the soup is at a gentle simmer.

Whisk the milk and flour together until creamy. Slowly pour the mixture into the pan, gently stirring to incorporate it. Heat until the soup is thickened, 2 to 3 minutes.

Per serving: 491.8 calories, 45.5 grams protein, 73 grams carbohydrates, 3.7 grams fat, 9.4 grams fiber

MAIN DISHES

Turkey, Fire-Roasted Pepper, and Spinach Salad

Spinach, carrots, roasted peppers, nuts, and cheese topped with grilled turkey in a great homemade dressing makes a perfect low-cal fat-burning meal.

MAKES 4 SERVINGS

½ cup low-sodium chicken broth

1 tablespoon extra-virgin olive oil

4 (4-ounce) skinless and boneless turkey breasts

6 cups loosely packed baby spinach leaves

2 tablespoons no-sugar-added orange juice

1 tablespoon apple cider vinegar

1 tablespoon extra-virgin olive oil

⅓ cup chopped raw, unsalted walnuts

2 teaspoons freshly squeezed lime juice

¼ teaspoon granulated garlic

¼ teaspoon chili powder

1 medium red bell pepper

¼ pound reduced-fat Feta cheese (or rice or soy cheese)

½ cup sliced carrots

½ small red onion, thinly sliced

Freshly ground black pepper

2 tablespoons minced fresh cilantro

Preheat the grill to high.

Combine the chicken broth and oil in a measuring cup. With the lid down, grill the turkey for about 1 hour, or until the center reaches 170°F, brushing with the broth mixture every 15 minutes and rotating once or twice. Set aside in a warm oven, covered, until ready to serve, but do not turn off the grill.

Place the spinach in a large bowl and set aside. Whisk together the orange juice, vinegar, and oil.

Heat a heavy-bottomed skillet over medium heat and toast the walnuts for 5 minutes, shaking the pan frequently. When the walnuts are golden brown, place them in a small bowl and immediately toss with the lime juice. Sprinkle on the garlic and chili powder, and toss to coat the nuts evenly.

Place the bell pepper directly on the grill at medium-high heat, turning it

MAIN DISHES

frequently until the skin is charred black all over, 10 to 15 minutes. Put the pepper in a paper bag, close the bag, and set it aside for a few minutes. When the pepper is cool enough to handle, rub off the skin, and cut the pepper in half. Discard the stem, seeds, and membranes, and cut the pepper into 1-inch-wide strips.

Add the cheese, carrots, onion, and orange juice mixture to the spinach, and toss well. Distribute equally among four chilled salad plates. Top each serving with equal amounts of bell pepper strips and spiced nuts. Grind a little black pepper on each one and sprinkle evenly with the cilantro.

Per serving: 338.8 calories, 43.2 grams protein, 9.3 grams carbohydrates, 14.8 grams fat, 3.7 grams fiber

MAIN DISHES

You don't have to run for the border to experience this tasty taco salad.

1 pound ground turkey or chicken breast

2 tablespoons extra-virgin olive oil

2 cups diced Roma tomatoes

1 (1.25-ounce) package taco seasoning mixed with water according to package
  directions

3 cups grated cabbage

1 cup loosely packed baby spinach leaves

½ cup plain nonfat Greek yogurt

½ cup prepared salsa

1 cup shredded Cheddar cheese (or rice or soy cheese)

4 tablespoons chopped green onion

Brown the turkey for 4 to 5 minutes in oil in large pan over medium-high heat. Stir in the tomatoes and taco seasoning mixture, and remove from the heat and drain off any excess liquid.

Combine the cabbage and spinach in a large salad bowl. Top with the turkey mixture, then the yogurt, salsa, and cheese. Sprinkle with the green onion and serve.

Per serving: 362 calories, 41 grams protein, 16 grams carbohydrates, 18 grams fat, 5 grams fiber

MAIN DISHES

Tropical Turkey Sausage and Shrimp Skewers

MAKES 4 SERVINGS

You'll imagine you're in the Bahamas when you enjoy these garlicky sausage and shrimp skewers.

2 (6-ounce) lean turkey sausages

2 cups fresh pineapple chunks

¾ pound peeled and deveined shrimp

¼ cup gold rum

2 tablespoons no-sugar-added orange juice

1 tablespoon extra-virgin olive oil

1 teaspoon minced gingerroot

1 teaspoon minced garlic

¼ teaspoon crushed red pepper flakes

¼ teaspoon dried marjoram

Soak 8 bamboo skewers in water for 30 minutes.

Cut the sausages into ¾-inch rounds, discarding the ends.

Thread equal portions of pineapple chunks, shrimp, and sausage slices alternately onto the skewers, and place them in a glass baking dish.

Combine the rum, orange juice, oil, ginger, garlic, red pepper, and marjoram in a small glass jar; cover tightly and shake to combine the ingredients. Pour over the kabobs, turning to coat them evenly. Cover and refrigerate for 1 hour, turning them occasionally.

Preheat the grill to medium.

Remove the kabobs from the marinade and place them on the grill rack. Cover the grill and cook the kabobs, turning them once or twice, until the sausages and shrimp are cooked through, about 10 minutes.

Per serving: 316.8 calories, 32.4 grams protein, 9.6 grams carbohydrates, 12.4 grams fat, 0.9 grams fiber

Grilled Sausage Pasta Salad

This hearty dish of turkey sausage, heart-healthy pasta, plump tomatoes, and eggplant is sure to become one of your favorite fat-burning meals.

MAKES 4 SERVINGS

5 tablespoons extra-virgin olive oil

6 tablespoons red wine vinegar

2 cloves garlic, minced

1 teaspoon dried oregano

½ teaspoon freshly ground black pepper

4 plum tomatoes, halved lengthwise

1 (1½-pound) eggplant, peeled and cut into ½-inch-thick slices

1 large red onion, cut into ½-inch-thick slices

2 turkey sausages

½ pound whole wheat wagon wheel pasta

Preheat the grill to medium-high. Coat the grill rack with nonstick cooking spray.

Whisk 4 tablespoons of the oil with the vinegar, garlic, oregano, and black pepper. Set aside.

Lightly coat the tomatoes, eggplant, and onion with the remaining 1 tablespoon of oil. Grill the vegetables and sausages, turning often, until the sausages are no longer pink and the vegetables are crisp-tender, 13 to 15 minutes.

Meanwhile, cook the pasta according to package directions. Drain and place in a large bowl.

Remove the vegetables from the grill and chop them into bite-size pieces. Cut the sausages into rounds, and then cut each round in half. Add the sausages, vegetables, and reserved dressing to the pasta, and toss to combine.

Per serving: 467.3 calories, 17.7 grams protein, 56.1 grams carbohydrates, 23.5 grams fat, 11.4 grams fiber

MAIN DISHES

**MAKES 4
SERVINGS**

Don't stress about eating pasta; just relax and enjoy!

¾ pound whole wheat fusilli

½ cup sliced carrots

½ cup asparagus cut into 1-inch pieces

½ cup broccoli florets

1 pound turkey sausage, cut into 1-inch pieces

2 cups grape or cherry tomatoes, halved

3 tablespoons chopped fresh basil

Freshly ground black pepper

Cook the fusilli according to package directions. During the last 3 minutes of cooking, add the carrots, asparagus, and broccoli to the pasta water. Drain and reserve ½ cup of the cooking water.

Heat a nonstick skillet over medium-high heat, and cook the sausage for 8 minutes. When it is almost cooked through, add the tomatoes and continue cooking 4 to 5 more minutes, or until the sausage is done.

Add the pasta and vegetables to the skillet with the sausage mixture. Then add the reserved cooking water and heat through. Stir in the basil, season with black pepper, and serve.

Per serving: 541.8 calories, 32.8 grams protein, 74 grams carbohydrates, 11.5 grams fat, 8.7 grams fiber

MAIN DISHES

Marinated Steak with Blue Cheese Topping

Steak and blue cheese is a classic combo and a great protein for your fat-burning meal.

MAKES 6
SERVINGS

½ cup red wine vinegar

½ cup extra-virgin olive oil

2 teaspoons dried thyme

1 clove garlic, chopped

1 teaspoon freshly ground black pepper

6 (4-ounce) rib-eye steaks

½ cup light butter, softened

½ cup stilton cheese, grated

2 teaspoons chopped fresh flat-leaf parsley

3 tablespoons chopped walnuts

Combine the vinegar, oil, thyme, garlic, and black pepper in a small bowl. Put the steaks in a baking dish and pour the vinegar mixture over them. Let the steaks marinate for 30 minutes at room temperature or for 3 hours in the refrigerator.

Meanwhile, in a small bowl, mash the butter and cheese with the parsley and walnuts until combined. Roll it up in wax paper to make a log shape and refrigerate until ready to serve the steaks.

Drain the marinade from the steaks and grill them at medium-high heat, about 5 minutes on each side or to your preferred doneness. Slice the stilton butter into 6 pats, and place 1 on each steak just before serving.

Per serving: 462.3 calories, 37.4 grams protein, 1.1 grams carbohydrates, 34.1 grams fat, 0.7 grams fiber

MAIN DISHES

MAKES 6 SERVINGS

Tired of a thousand-calorie burger blowing up your meal? Try this healthier version instead.

1 egg white, slightly beaten

2 tablespoons water

¼ cup whole wheat bread crumbs

¼ cup finely shredded carrot

¼ cup finely chopped onion

¼ cup finely chopped red bell pepper

⅛ teaspoon freshly ground black pepper

2 tablespoons freshly grated Parmesan cheese (or rice or soy cheese)

1 pound lean ground beef

6 whole wheat buns

12 lettuce leaves

6 tomato slices

12 red onion slices

In a large bowl, combine the egg white, water, bread crumbs, carrot, onion, bell pepper, and black pepper. Add the cheese and beef, and mix well. Shape into six ½-inch-thick patties.

Spray a grill pan with non-stick cooking spray and cook the burgers for 7 minutes over medium heat. Turn and cook until cooked through, 8 to 11 minutes more.

Serve the burgers on buns, each with 2 lettuce leaves, 1 tomato slice, and 2 onion slices.

Per serving: 320.5 calories, 23 grams protein, 31.2 grams carbohydrates, 13.7 grams fat, 6.3 gram fiber

MAIN DISHES

Sliced Steak Salad with Chutney

This spicy, crunchy steak salad will keep you on the road to a lean and healthy life!

MAKES 4
SERVINGS

4 (4-ounce) sirloin steaks

4 teaspoons lemon pepper

2 teaspoons minced garlic

1 large Vidalia onion, sliced

1 tablespoon extra-virgin olive oil

8 cups spinach leaves, stemmed

1 (10-ounce) package frozen asparagus, cooked and chilled

1 cup plain whole wheat croutons

½ cup prepared vinaigrette dressing

⅓ cup chutney

Preheat the grill to high.

Sprinkle the steaks with the lemon pepper and garlic.

Grill for about 3 minutes per side or until done to your liking. Let stand for 5 minutes before slicing them diagonally across the grain. Brush the onion slices with the oil and grill on medium heat until tender, about 3 minutes.

Divide the spinach among four plates. Top with equal portions of asparagus, grilled onion, and croutons. Add 1 sliced steak to each plate, and drizzle each with 2 tablespoons of the vinaigrette and 4 teaspoons of the chutney.

Per serving: 408.8 calories, 41.2 grams protein, 33.3 grams carbohydrates, 12.2 grams fat, 5.1 grams fiber

MAIN DISHES

MAKES 6 SERVINGS

Serve this salsa-topped steak with steamed veggies and a baked potato to make a complete fat-burning meal.

6 (4-ounce) sirloin steaks

⅓ cup light Italian dressing

6 tablespoons freshly squeezed lime juice

2 tablespoons minced garlic

1 tablespoon Greek seasoning*

1 cup chopped tomato

1 teaspoon finely chopped jalapeño pepper

¼ cup peeled and chopped cucumber

4 (½-inch-thick) fresh pineapple slices

6 lemon slices

Place the steaks in a large sealable plastic bag.

In a bowl, combine the Italian dressing, lime juice, garlic, and Greek seasoning. Pour the marinade over the steaks. Seal the bag and shake well. Refrigerate for 2 hours.

In a bowl, combine the tomato, jalapeño, and cucumber. Cover and refrigerate along with the steaks.

Preheat the grill to medium-high. Coat the grill rack with nonstick cooking spray. Grill the pineapple and lemon slices until grill marks appear, 3 to 4 minutes on each side. Remove from the heat and set aside.

Remove the steaks from the marinade, discard the marinade, and grill the steaks on medium-high heat for 6 to 8 minutes on each side or to preferred doneness.

Remove and discard the peel from the lemon slices. Chop the lemon and pineapple, and stir into the tomato mixture.

Serve the steaks, topping each with ⅓ to ½ cup of the salsa.

Per serving: 255.7 calories, 35 grams protein, 9.3 grams carbohydrates, 8.4 grams fat, 1 gram fiber

---

*Greek seasoning is available in the spice aisle of most supermarkets.

MAIN DISHES

Imagine you're in Hawaii when you enjoy these steak and pineapple kebabs.

For the marinade

½ cup tequila

2 teaspoons extra-virgin olive oil

4 tablespoons freshly squeezed lime juice

¼ cup hoisin sauce

4 cloves garlic, minced

Juice from 1 (20-ounce) can pineapple chunks (reserve the fruit for the kabobs)

For the kabobs

2 pounds sirloin steak, cut into 1-inch cubes

1 red bell pepper, cored, seeded, and cut into 1-inch chunks

1 green bell pepper, cored, seeded, and cut into 1-inch chunks

1 large onion, cut into 1-inch cubes

1 (20-ounce) can pineapple chunks, drained (reserve the juice)

2 limes, cut into ¼-inch-thick slices

Soak 12 bamboo skewers in water for 30 minutes.

Make the marinade: Place all the marinade ingredients in a large bowl and mix well. Add the steak cubes and marinate in the refrigerator for at least 1 hour.

Preheat the grill to medium.

Evenly distribute the bell peppers, onions, pineapple, and steak onto the skewers, placing a slice of lime on one or both sides of each cube of steak. Reserve the marinade. Grill for 5 minutes per side, turning once. Drizzle the reserved marinade over the kabobs after turning. Remove the skewers and discard the lime slices before serving.

Per serving: 454.2 calories, 47 grams protein, 27.7 grams carbohydrates, 11.6 grams fat, 1.9 grams fiber

MAIN DISHES

MAKES 6 SERVINGS

Grilled steak, tender vegetables, and melted cheese combine to make one fun-in-the-sun Greek-style pizza.

For the crust

2 cups whole wheat flour

1 package active dry yeast or instant yeast

1 cup hot tap water (120°F–125°F)

1 tablespoon extra-virgin olive oil

1 tablespoon honey (organic if possible) or granulated sugar

For the topping

1 pound lean steak

Freshly ground black pepper

2 cups grape tomatoes

1 cup pitted and chopped kalamata olives

1 tablespoon dried oregano

2 tablespoons extra-virgin olive oil

1 large eggplant, peeled and cut into ½-inch-thick slices

1 cup prepared sun-dried tomato pesto

½ pound shredded fat-free mozzarella cheese (or rice or soy cheese)

½ pound low-fat Feta cheese (or rice or soy cheese), crumbled

1 tablespoon chopped fresh cilantro

Make the crust: In large mixing bowl, combine the flour and yeast. Stir in the water, oil, and honey. Mix by hand until all the ingredients are well mixed, about 3 minutes. Cover with plastic wrap and set aside to rise until doubled, 2 to 3 hours at most.

Preheat the oven to 425°F. Spray a 12- to 14-inch pizza pan with nonstick cooking spray.

Transfer the dough to the prepared pan and press it down, covering the bottom of the pan and going up the sides to form a rim.

Bake for 15 to 20 minutes, or until the crust is golden brown. Remove the pan from the oven and lower the heat to 375°F.

Make the topping: Preheat the grill to high.

Season the steak with black pepper and grill on medium heat for about 7 minutes on each side or to your preferred degree of doneness. Toss the tomatoes, olives, oregano, and 1 tablespoon of the oil in a mixing bowl. Spread the mixture on a baking sheet in one even layer. Roast in the oven for 15 minutes, or until the tomatoes begin to blister and pop.

Coat the eggplant with the remaining 1 tablespoon of oil. Grill until browned and tender, 5 minutes on each side. Remove and let cool, then cut into cubes and set aside.

Grill pizza crust for 1 minute, then flip it over and turn the grill on low. Remove pizza crust from grill and top with the pesto, mozzarella, tomato mixture, eggplant, steak, Feta cheese, and cilantro. Return pizza to the grill and close the lid, cooking just until the cheese is melted. Lift gently from time to time to check the bottom of the crust. If it is getting burned, turn off the heat and leave the lid closed until the cheese is melted.

Remove from the heat and set aside for 5 minutes before cutting into 6 wedges.

Per serving: 532.2 calories, 40.3 grams protein, 48.6 grams carbohydrates, 19.3 grams fat, 8.6 grams fiber

MAIN DISHES

Venison Stew

Close to nature and lean on the hips, venison stew offers a perfect balance of protein and carbs.

1 tablespoon extra-virgin olive oil

1 pound venison, cubed

½ cup chopped onion

2 cups low-sodium beef broth

⅔ cup uncooked barley

½ teaspoon dried oregano

¼ teaspoon freshly ground black pepper

1 (16-ounce) can whole tomatoes with their liquid

1 (16-ounce) package frozen mixed vegetables

1 tablespoon minced garlic

Add the oil to a large stockpot and heat over medium heat. Add the venison and onion, and cook until brown.

Add the remaining ingredients to the pot, cover, and simmer over medium to low heat until meat is tender, 1½ to 2 hours.

Per serving: 368.6 calories, 41.3 grams protein, 41.5 grams carbohydrates, 4.4 grams fat, 6.6 grams fiber

MAIN DISHES

This combination of halibut, sugar snap peas, and baby carrots accompanied by couscous makes a complete fat-burning meal. You can even add a green salad if you like.

¾ cup peeled baby carrots

2 small zucchinis or yellow summer squash, halved lengthwise
    and cut crosswise into ½-inch-thick slices

1½ pounds halibut fillets, cut into 1-inch cubes

1 cup fresh sugar snap peas, topped and tailed

1 teaspoon ground cumin

1 teaspoon ground coriander

¼ teaspoon freshly ground black pepper

¼ teaspoon cayenne pepper

3 tablespoons extra-virgin olive oil

¼ cup freshly squeezed orange juice

1 cup quick-cooking couscous

1 teaspoon finely grated orange zest

1½ cups low-sodium chicken broth

Soak 6 bamboo skewers in water for 30 minutes.

Bring 6 cups of water to a boil in a medium saucepan, add the carrots, and cook over medium heat for 1 minute. Add the zucchini and cook 1 minute more. Drain and set aside.

Thread the halibut, squash, carrots, and sugar snap peas onto the skewers, leaving a ¼-inch space between the pieces.

In a small bowl, stir together the cumin, coriander, black pepper, and cayenne. In a medium saucepan, heat the oil over low heat. Add the spice mixture and stir for 1 minute. Transfer 2 tablespoons of the spice mixture to a small bowl and whisk in the orange juice.

Add the couscous to the saucepan and stir until coated. Cook and stir for 1 minute, then add the orange zest and broth. Bring to a boil; cover and remove from the heat; and let stand, covered, until ready to serve.

MAIN DISHES

Brush the kebabs with half the orange juice mixture. Spray a grill pan with nonstick cooking spray and place it over medium heat. Grill the kebabs until the fish flakes easily with a fork, about 10 minutes. Halfway through grilling, turn and brush with the remaining orange juice mixture. Serve with the couscous.

Per serving: 318.5 calories, 29.4 grams protein, 29 grams carbohydrates, 10.1 grams fat, 4.9 grams fiber

Lemony Salmon with Couscous and String Beans

Here's a satisfying fat-burning meal for any season of the year.

2 lemons, sliced into thin rounds

4 (4-ounce) salmon steaks, skin removed

2 tablespoons freshly squeezed lemon juice

1½ teaspoons freshly ground black pepper

4 large sprigs fresh rosemary

2 tablespoons light butter

1 cup cooked whole wheat couscous

4 cups steamed string beans

Preheat the grill to medium.

Tear off four squares of aluminum foil, each four times larger than a salmon steak. Line each aluminum foil square with enough lemon slices to cover the bottom of a salmon steak.

Put a salmon steak on the lemons, and pour one-quarter of the lemon juice over each. Sprinkle with black pepper, place a sprig of rosemary on each steak, and top each one with ½ tablespoon of the butter.

Bring the ends of the aluminum foil up over the salmon and fold them over to seal. Then bring up the ends to make a sealed packet.

Grill the salmon for about 10 minutes, turn, and cook 5 to 10 minutes more, until cooked through. Open the packets carefully and check to ensure salmon is done to your likeness; the steam will be hot. If not done, return to the grill and check every 2 to 3 minutes.

Serve each salmon steak with ¼ cup of couscous and 1 cup of string beans.

Per serving: 481 calories, 34.6 grams protein, 50.5 grams carbohydrates, 17.5 grams fat, 10.5 grams fiber

MAIN DISHES

MAKES 4 SERVINGS

This fruit-topped salmon dish is an ideal protein for any fat-burning meal.

For the salsa

⅓ cup blueberries

⅓ cup peeled, diced mango

2 tablespoons minced red onion

2 tablespoons minced red bell pepper

1 tablespoon minced fresh cilantro

1 tablespoon freshly squeezed lime juice

½ teaspoon seeded and minced jalapeño pepper

2 teaspoons evaporated cane juice (see note on page 145)

For the salmon

1 tablespoon extra-virgin olive oil

4 (4-ounce) salmon fillets

Pinch of freshly ground black pepper

Make the salsa: Combine all the salsa ingredients in a medium bowl. Press lightly with the back of a spoon to release the juices from the fruit and set aside.

Make the salmon: Heat the oil in a large skillet over medium-high heat. Season the salmon with pepper and sear it until it is cooked through, 3 to 5 minutes per side.

Serve the fillets topped with the salsa.

Per serving: 261.8 calories, 22.7 grams protein, 10.3 grams carbohydrates, 3.9 grams fat, 0.5 grams fiber)

MAIN DISHES

This combination may sound odd, but it's really very tasty, so try it. I bet you'll like it.

1 medium yam

1 (6-ounce) can water-packed Albacore tuna

Freshly ground black pepper

Mustard

Use a fork to poke holes in the yam and microwave it on high for 6 to 7 minutes.

Cube the yam flesh and measure 1 cup of cubes. Transfer to a dinner plate, top with the tuna, add pepper and mustard to taste, and serve.

Per serving: 395 calories, 42.3 grams protein, 41.8 grams carbohydrates, 5.4 grams fat, 6 grams fiber

MAIN DISHES

The fish of your choice smothered in Chinese flavors makes for a great protein to go with ½ cup steamed rice for women, ⅔ cup for men, and a portion of grilled veggies.

1 (18- to 20-inch-long) whole lake trout, salmon, or similar fish

3 tablespoons low-sodium soy sauce

3 tablespoons hoisin sauce

2 tablespoons black bean sauce with garlic*

1 tablespoon sesame oil

1 tablespoon dry sherry

1 teaspoon finely minced fresh gingerroot

Rinse the fish inside and out, and pat dry. Make deep slashes through the skin about 2 inches apart on both sides and parallel with the gills. You will have 4 to 5 slashes per side.

Tear off a piece of heavy-duty foil 4 inches longer than the fish. Fold it in half lengthwise, and turn up the edges to form a shallow rim. Place the foil on a baking sheet, and place the fish on the foil.

In a small bowl, mix together all the remaining ingredients. Pour a quarter of the mixture over one side of the fish and rub it into the slits with your fingers. Turn the fish over and pour a similar amount of the mixture over the other side, rubbing it into the slits. Reserve the remaining mixture. Cover and refrigerate the fish for at least 15 minutes or up to 2 hours.

Preheat the grill to medium.

Carefully lift the foil-cradled fish onto the grill grate. Pour half the remaining soy sauce mixture over the fish. Cover the grill and cook for 15 minutes. Pour the remaining soy sauce mixture over the fish; re-cover the grill, and cook for 10 minutes longer.

Carefully pull the foil-cradled fish to the side of the grill so that the back part

*This sauce is generally available at Asian groceries and markets. If you can't find this sauce, mash whole black beans to an equal amount and combine them with fresh garlic to taste.

Diet-Free for Life

of the fish is still partially over the heat; the belly side should not be over the hot area. Re-cover the grill and cook an additional 5 minutes or until the fish is cooked through.

Per serving: 267.8 calories, 21.8 grams protein, 9 grams carbohydrates, 15.5 grams fat, 0.8 grams fiber

Fish-Stuffed Peppers

Add a fast carb to this fish dish for a complete fat-burning meal.

2 tablespoons drained capers

½ cup light mayonnaise

2 teaspoons snipped fresh dill

2 teaspoons Dijon mustard

1 pound skinless and boneless fish fillets, cut into ½-inch cubes

2 green bell peppers

1 teaspoon extra-virgin olive oil

2 tablespoons whole wheat bread crumbs

2 tablespoons light butter, melted

Preheat the grill to medium-high.

In a medium bowl, mash the capers slightly with a fork. Add the mayonnaise, dill, and mustard, and stir to mix well. Add the fish; stir gently to blend. Set aside.

Keeping the peppers whole, carefully cut off the tops and remove the seeds and membranes, leaving as much of the flesh as possible.

Brush the insides with the oil and place the peppers, cut side up, on the grill grate directly over the heat. Grill until the pepper skins have colored in spots and the peppers are somewhat soft, about 5 minutes.

Transfer the peppers to a plate, but do not turn off the grill. Stuff the peppers with equal amounts of the fish mixture. In a small bowl, toss the bread crumbs with the melted butter and sprinkle the mixture over the fish.

Return the peppers to the grill but not directly over the heat. Cover the grill and cook for 25 minutes. The crumb mixture should be golden and the fish cooked through.

Lay the cooked peppers on their sides and carefully cut them in half horizontally. Serve a half of stuffed pepper per person.

Per serving: 220.3 calories, 22.1 grams protein, 11.7 grams carbohydrates, 9.6 grams fat, 1.8 grams fiber

MAIN DISHES

If you are ever in the mood for Mexican flavor, this fat-burning meal is right for you. Low-carb soft tacos and tilapia fillets will send your taste buds on a tropical vacation.

- 1 tablespoon extra-virgin olive oil
- 1 pound tilapia fillets
- ½ cup plain nonfat Greek yogurt
- 2 tablespoons freshly squeezed lime juice
- 4 low-carb whole wheat tortillas
- 1 cup shredded green cabbage
- ½ cup prepared salsa

Coat a frying pan with the oil, and set it over medium heat. Cook the tilapia fillets until opaque and flaky, about 7 minutes on each side.

Meanwhile, in a small bowl, whisk together the yogurt and lime juice. To assemble the tacos, divide the cooked fish among the tortillas and top with equal portions of cabbage, yogurt sauce, and salsa.

Per serving: 430.5 calories, 62.7 grams protein, 27.1 grams carbohydrates, 14.3 grams fat, 13.9 grams fiber

MAIN DISHES

Fresh Fish Stew

This waistline-friendly stew combines slow carbs and protein. Serve it with crusty bread and a green salad to make a complete fat-burning meal.

3 cloves garlic, diced

¾ cup chopped onion

2 tablespoons water

1 medium green bell pepper, cored, seeded, and cut into 1-inch strips

2 medium carrots, cut into ½-inch rounds

3 celery stalks, cut into 1-inch pieces

2 cups diced red potatoes, peeled

1 (15-ounce) can no-salt-added tomato sauce

1 (15-ounce) can no-salt-added diced tomatoes with their liquid*

1½ tablespoons honey (organic if possible)

½ teaspoon ground thyme

⅛ teaspoon cayenne pepper (optional)

1 bay leaf

½ pound halibut, cut into bite-size pieces

½ pound salmon, cut into bite-size pieces

¼ cup chopped fresh flat-leaf parsley

Lemon wedges, balsamic vinegar, or red wine vinegar for serving

Combine the garlic, onion, and water in a stockpot.

Cook over medium heat until the onion softens and the liquid evaporates, 3 to 5 minutes.

Add the green pepper, carrots, celery, potatoes, tomato sauce, tomatoes and their liquid, honey, thyme, cayenne pepper (if using), and bay leaf.

Bring to a boil, cover, and simmer 50 minutes, or until the potatoes are tender.

Add the fish to the pot and cook, uncovered, until cooked through, about 8 minutes.

Sprinkle with the parsley and serve with lemon wedges or vinegar.

Per serving: 373 calories, 33 grams protein, 41.9 grams carbohydrates, 9.3 grams fat, 6.8 grams fiber

---

*If the tomatoes are whole, crush them with the back of a spoon once you add them to the pot.

MAIN DISHES

Add your favorite fast carb to these swordfish and tomato skewers to make a fat-burning meal for a family of four.

For the pesto

1 cup fresh cilantro leaves

½ cup fresh mint leaves

3 tablespoons freshly squeezed orange juice

2 tablespoons chopped green onion

1 tablespoon freshly squeezed lime juice

2 teaspoons extra-virgin olive oil

1 clove garlic

For the skewers

2 teaspoons grated lime zest

1 teaspoon grated orange zest

1 tablespoon freshly squeezed lime juice

2 tablespoons freshly squeezed orange juice

2 teaspoons evaporated cane juice (see note on page 145)

2 cloves garlic, minced

1½ pounds swordfish fillets cut into 1¼-inch cubes

24 cherry tomatoes

¼ teaspoon freshly ground black pepper

Make the pesto: Combine all the ingredients in a food processor and process until smooth. Set aside while you prepare the fish.

Make skewers: Combine the lime and orange zests, lime and orange juices, cane juice, and garlic in a large sealable plastic bag. Add the fish and seal the bag. Marinate in the refrigerator for 30 minutes, turning the bag once.

Soak 8 bamboo skewers in water for 30 minutes. Preheat the grill to medium-high.

Remove the fish from the bag and discard the marinade. Thread the fish and tomatoes equally onto the skewers, and season with the black pepper.

MAIN DISHES

Place skewers on a grill rack coated with cooking spray, turning every 2 minutes for about 6 minutes, or until your preferred doneness.

Serve with the pesto.

Per serving: 279.5 calories, 35.2 grams protein, 13.5 grams carbohydrates, 10.3 grams fat, 1.8 grams fiber

This is my version of a delicious Vietnamese-style dish combing shrimp, mango, and avocado. Add rice or any other fast carb for a perfect fat-burning meal.

MAKES 6 SERVINGS

¾ cup water

1 tablespoon Splenda

6 tablespoons freshly squeezed lime juice

2½ tablespoons fish sauce

1 clove garlic, minced

1 tablespoon finely grated carrot

1 tablespoon thinly sliced serrano pepper (about 1 pepper)

36 large shrimp, peeled and butterflied, tails intact

2 ripe unpeeled avocados, halved and pitted

2 peeled mangoes, each cut into 6 wedges

12 lime wedges

6 large Bibb lettuce leaves

Chopped fresh cilantro (optional)

Soak 12 bamboo skewers in water for 30 minutes.

Combine the water, Splenda, lime juice, fish sauce, and garlic in a small bowl. Remove and reserve ¾ cup of the mixture. Stir the carrot and serrano pepper into what remains in the bowl.

In a large bowl, combine the shrimp with the reserved juice mixture, tossing to coat well. Cover and refrigerate, letting the shrimp marinate for 1 hour, tossing them occasionally. Remove the shrimp from the bowl, but do not discard the marinade.

Preheat the grill to medium-high.

Place the marinade in a small saucepan and bring to a boil. Lower the heat and simmer 5 minutes.

Place 3 shrimp on each skewer. Put the shrimp on a grill rack coated with nonstick cooking spray and grill until done, brushing frequently with the cooked marinade, 2½ minutes on each side.

MAIN DISHES

Cut 3 avocado halves in half lengthwise. Peel and dice the remaining half and set aside. Brush the cooked marinade over the mango wedges and avocado quarters, and coat with cooking spray. Arrange on the grill rack with the lime wedges and grill until marked but not soft, brushing frequently with the cooked marinade, 2 minutes on each side.

Place a lettuce leaf on each of 6 plates; top each with 1 mango wedge, 1 avocado quarter, and 2 lime wedges. Place 2 skewers of shrimp on each plate; sprinkle with the diced avocado and cilantro, if using, and serve with the reserved juice mixture.

Per serving: 346 calories, 15.9 grams protein, 34.7 grams carbohydrates, 16.5 grams fat, 9.9 grams fiber

Charleston Shrimp and Grits

When combined with a protein, grits (or hominy) makes for a quick, tasty, and delicious fat-burning meal! Although grits are sometimes underappreciated outside the South, this recipe is a great introduction to why they are so loved from Louisiana to the Carolinas.

1½ pounds medium shrimp, peeled, halved lengthwise, and deveined

2 tablespoons freshly squeezed lemon juice

Hot pepper sauce

6 cups water

1½ cups stone-ground grits (not instant or quick-cooking)

2 tablespoons light butter

1 small onion, finely chopped (optional)

¼ cup finely chopped green bell pepper

1 clove garlic, minced

½ cup thinly sliced green onions

2 tablespoons unbleached all-purpose flour

1 cup low-sodium vegetable or chicken stock

1 cup grated medium to sharp low-fat Cheddar cheese (or rice or soy cheese)

Combine the shrimp with 1 tablespoon of the lemon juice and a couple of generous splashes of hot sauce. Set aside.

Bring the water to a boil in a large heavy saucepan over medium-high heat. Whisk in the grits a few handfuls at a time. (They will bubble up initially.) When you have added all the grits, reduce the heat to low and simmer very slowly for 35 to 40 minutes, stirring occasionally at first and more frequently toward the end.

Meanwhile, melt 1 tablespoon of the butter in a medium pan over medium heat. Stir in the onion (if using), bell pepper, and garlic. Cook until the onion and pepper are limp, about 5 minutes. Add the green onion, sprinkle the flour over the mixture, and continue to cook and stir for 5 minutes longer. Stir in the stock and cook for 5 minutes longer. Remove from the heat while you finish the grits.

MAIN DISHES

When the grits are thick and creamy, stir in the remaining 1 tablespoon of butter followed by the cheese. Add a splash of hot sauce to taste. Remove from the heat and cover.

Return the gravy to medium heat and stir in the shrimp. Cook until the shrimp are opaque throughout, about 5 minutes. Serve immediately, mounding the grits in large shallow bowls or on plates, and covering them with shrimp and gravy. Sprinkle with the remaining lemon juice.

Per serving: 343 calories, 45.9 grams protein, 22.9 grams carbohydrates, 6.8 grams fat, 1.3 grams fiber

A splash of tequila, lime, and cilantro puts a little kick in these shrimp tacos.

2 tablespoons extra-virgin olive oil

1 large yellow onion, finely chopped

½ to 1 jalapeño pepper, seeded and minced

2 cloves garlic

1 pound medium shrimp, peeled, deveined, and cut into small pieces

¼ cup tequila

2 tablespoons freshly squeezed lime juice

6 low-carb whole wheat or corn tortillas

1 avocado, sliced

3 cups shredded green cabbage

¼ cup chopped fresh cilantro

1 cup mild white cheese (or rice or soy cheese), grated

Salad dressing of your choice

Heat the oil in a large frying pan over medium heat. Add the onion, jalapeño pepper, and garlic, and sauté until lightly browned.

Add the shrimp and tequila, and continue cooking until the shrimp are opaque. Sprinkle the lime juice over the shrimp mixture, stir, and remove from the heat.

Heat the tortillas in a dry pan over medium heat until lightly crunchy.

Divide the shrimp and onion mixture evenly over each tortilla. Divide the avocado, cabbage, cilantro, and cheese over top, and pour a small amount of dressing on each serving.

Per serving: 570.8 calories, 59.4 grams protein, 47.7 grams carbohydrates, 24.3 grams fat, 27.8 grams fiber

MAIN DISHES

Black Bean and Cheese Burrito

The softness of the tortilla combines with the warmth of the beans and the melted goodness of the cheese to create a delicious fat-burning meal. Serve with a large salad topped with Fat-Burning Salad Dressing (see page 213).

1 large low-carb, low-fat tortilla

1 cup canned black beans

¼ cup shredded soy Cheddar-style cheese

Spray a large skillet with nonstick cooking spray. Lay the tortilla in the skillet and cook over medium heat until lightly browned.

Meanwhile, heat the beans in a saucepan over medium heat.

Transfer the tortilla to a serving plate, top with the beans and cheese, roll up, and serve.

Per serving: 375 calories, 30.5 grams protein, 55 grams carbohydrates, 8.5 grams fat, 25.5 grams fiber

Broiled Eggplant and Mozzarella with Tomato and Basil ⓥ

MAKES 2
SERVINGS

Grilled eggplant stuffed with ripe tomatoes, melted mozzarella, and fresh basil provides any diet-free vegetarian with a great lunch. Serve with a large salad with 1 cup of slow-carb veggies or 1 slice of your preferred bread.

1 large eggplant

2 tablespoons extra-virgin olive oil

⅜ pound soy mozzarella-style cheese, cut into 8 slices

2 plum tomatoes, each cut into 4 slices

8 large basil leaves

Freshly ground black pepper

Balsamic vinegar, for drizzling (optional)

Preheat the broiler and line a broiler pan with foil.

Cut and peel the eggplant lengthwise into 10 equal slices, discarding the 2 outermost slices. Rinse and pat dry.

Place the eggplant slices in the pan and brush with the oil. Broil for 4 to 5 minutes until golden and tender. Turn and brush with more oil, broiling for 4 to 5 more minutes.

Remove the eggplant from the broiler. In the middle of each eggplant slice, place 1 slice of mozzarella, 1 tomato slice, and 1 basil leaf. Season with black pepper. Fold the eggplant over the filling and return to the broiler, seam-side down, until the filling is heated through and the cheese begins to melt.

Serve with a drizzle of balsamic, if using.

Per serving: 345 calories, 23.9 grams protein, 21.7 grams carbohydrates, 20 grams fat, 11.6 grams fiber

VEGETARIAN MAIN DISHES

**MAKES 1
SERVING**

By adding ripe tomatoes and a side of beans to your grilled cheese sandwich, you'll be creating a filling fat-burning meal.

1 cup black beans, rinsed and drained

1 tablespoon light butter

2 slices whole wheat bread

1 (1-ounce) slice low-fat mozzarella cheese (or rice or soy cheese)

3 (¼-inch-thick) slices tomato

Place the beans in a small saucepan over medium-low heat until warmed through.

Coat a pan with nonstick cooking spray and set it over medium-high heat. Spread butter on one side of each piece of bread. Place cheese and tomatoes on the unbuttered side of one slice; top with the second slice, buttered side up; and grill in the pan, turning once, until the bread is golden and the cheese is melted. Serve beans on the side.

Per serving: 430 calories, 23 grams protein, 55.7 grams carbohydrates, 13.5 grams fat, 11.2 grams fiber

VEGETARIAN MAIN DISHES

Egg whites combined with fresh bell pepper, onion, and garlic, accompanied by a toasted English muffin and a cup of orange juice, is a breakfast designed to meet the standards of any diet-free vegetarian.

MAKES 2 SERVINGS

1 tablespoon extra-virgin olive oil

½ onion, chopped (optional)

1 red bell pepper, cored, seeded, and thinly sliced

1 green bell pepper, cored, seeded, and thinly sliced

1 clove garlic, crushed

Freshly ground black pepper

6 large egg whites, beaten with 1 tablespoon water

2 (100% whole wheat) English muffins

1 cup unsweetened orange juice

Heat the oil in a large frying pan over medium heat. Add the onion, if using, and sauté until softened.

Add the bell peppers and cook another 5 minutes. Add the garlic, season with black pepper, and cook for another 5 minutes.

Pour the egg whites over the vegetables and cook, stirring occasionally, until the mixture has a consistency of scrambled eggs, 2 to 3 minutes.

Divide the eggs equally between two plates, and serve each portion with 1 English muffin (toasted, if preferred) and ½ cup of the orange juice.

Per serving: 333.5 calories, 18.2 grams protein, 47.3 grams carbohydrates, 9 grams fat, 6.6 grams fiber

VEGETARIAN MAIN DISHES

Pasta with Fresh Feta and Artichokes

The mixture of tender artichokes and whole wheat pasta topped with lightly melted cheese is a great vegetarian fat-burning meal to share with friends and family.

¾ pound whole wheat penne pasta

4 cups water

3 tablespoons freshly squeezed lemon juice

4 medium artichokes

2 tablespoons extra-virgin olive oil

2 tablespoons chopped garlic

¼ cup chopped fresh flat-leaf parsley

½ teaspoon freshly ground black pepper

½ cup soy cheese, diced

¾ cup low-fat Feta cheese (or rice or soy cheese)

Cook the pasta according to package directions without adding salt or fat. Drain and reserve ½ cup of the cooking water.

Meanwhile, combine the water and lemon juice. Trim and peel the stems of the artichokes leaving 1 inch. Remove the hard outer leaves, leaving only the tender hearts attached to the stems. Cut the artichokes in half lengthwise and remove the fuzzy thistle with a spoon. Cut the artichoke halves lengthwise into thin slices, placing them in the lemon water to prevent discoloration.

Heat the oil in a skillet over medium heat. Add the garlic and cook 1 minute. Remove the artichokes from the water and add to the skillet. Cover and cook, stirring occasionally, until the artichokes are tender, about 10 minutes.

In a large bowl, combine the artichoke mixture with the pasta, reserved cooking water, the parsley, and black pepper. Toss well and gently stir in the soy cheese a spoonful at a time. Spoon 1⅓ cup of the pasta mixture into each of 6 bowls, and top each serving with 2 tablespoons of Feta cheese.

Per serving: 340.8 calories, 16 grams protein, 54 grams carbohydrates, 8.6 grams fat, 10.4 grams fiber

VEGETARIAN MAIN DISHES

This simple-to-assemble vegetarian lasagna is stuffed with mushrooms and tomatoes to create a perfect fat-burning meal. Serve it with a side salad.

MAKES 5 SERVINGS

- ⅔ cup dried porcini mushrooms
- 2 tablespoons extra-virgin olive oil
- 1 large clove garlic, chopped
- 5 cups mixed fresh mushrooms, including brown cap, shiitake, and wild varieties, roughly sliced
- 10 fresh whole wheat lasagna sheets
- ¾ cup dry white wine
- 6 tablespoons chopped canned tomatoes
- ½ teaspoon evaporated cane juice (see note on page 145)
- ½ cup freshly grated low-fat Parmesan cheese (or rice or soy cheese)
- Freshly ground black pepper
- Fresh basil leaves, for garnish

Place the porcini mushrooms in a bowl and cover with boiling water. Leave to soak for 15 minutes, then drain and rinse.

Heat the oil in a large frying pan over medium heat, and sauté the porcinis over high heat until the edges are slightly crisp, about 5 minutes. Reduce the heat to medium; add the garlic and fresh mushrooms, and sauté until tender, about 5 minutes.

Meanwhile, without adding any extra fat, cook the lasagna according to package directions until it is al dente. Drain lightly; the pasta should still be moist.

Add the wine to the mushroom mixture and cook until the liquid is reduced, 5 to 7 minutes. Stir in the tomatoes and cane juice, and cook for 5 minutes.

Divide half of the sauce equally among 5 serving plates, place 1 lasagna sheet on top, and spoon the remaining sauce evenly over each serving. Top each with another lasagna sheet, and sprinkle each serving with 2 tablespoons of the cheese. Season with black pepper, and garnish with the basil leaves.

Per serving: 363.9 calories, 17 grams protein, 44.8 grams carbohydrates, 12 grams fat, 6.2 grams fiber

VEGETARIAN MAIN DISHES

**MAKES 4
SERVINGS**

The Mexican-style rice blended with tomatoes, carrots, onions, and beans and served with a warm low-carb tortilla provides enough fiber to cancel out the carbs in this delectable vegetarian fat-burning meal.

For the rice

4 tomatoes, halved and seeded

1 onion, sliced (optional)

2 clove garlic, chopped

2 tablespoons extra-virgin olive oil

1 cup uncooked long grain brown rice, rinsed

2½ cups vegetable stock

½ cup canned kidney beans, rinsed and drained

¾ cup fresh green beans, cut

2 carrots, diced

Freshly ground black pepper

For the salsa

1 avocado

2 tablespoons freshly squeezed lime juice

1 small red onion, diced

1 small red hot pepper, seeded and chopped

2 tablespoons canned kidney beans, rinsed and drained

Chopped fresh cilantro (optional)

8 low-carb tortillas

Make the rice: Heat the broiler to high. Spread the tomatoes, onion (if using), and garlic on a baking sheet, and coat with 1 tablespoon of the oil. Broil for 5 minutes and turn the vegetables over. Then broil another 5 minutes, or until the vegetables are softened. Set aside to cool.

Heat the remaining 1 tablespoon oil in a saucepan over medium heat, add the rice, and cook, stirring until golden brown, about 2 minutes.

In a food processor or blender, puree the broiled vegetables and stir them into the rice. Cook another 2 minutes, stirring frequently. Add the stock and cook for 20 minutes, stirring occasionally.

VEGETARIAN MAIN DISHES

Add the kidney beans, green beans, and carrots to the rice mixture. Cook until the vegetables are tender, about 15 minutes. Season with black pepper. Remove from the heat and let stand for 15 minutes.

Make the salsa: Pit, peel, and dice the avocado, and place it in a medium bowl. Squeeze in the lime juice and toss to coat. Mix in the onion, red pepper, kidney beans, and cilantro, if using.

Lay the tortillas in a skillet and warm over medium heat. To serve, divide the rice mixture equally among 4 plates and serve with 2 tortillas and a dollop of salsa.

Per serving: 398 calories, 21.5 grams protein, 57.3 grams carbohydrates, 18.3 grams fat, 22.8 grams fiber

Parmecharmed Pasta and Bean Soup

This is a complete vegetarian fat-burning meal. It combines hearty vegetables, beans, pasta, and a dash of spice to make it nice.

5 tablespoons extra-virgin olive oil

1 onion, chopped

1 celery stalk, chopped

2 carrots, chopped

1 bay leaf

5 cups low-sodium vegetable stock

3 cups chopped canned tomatoes

1½ cups small whole wheat pasta (such as farfalle or conchiglie)

3 cups canned borlotti or cannellini beans, rinsed and drained

8 cups spinach leaves, stemmed and chopped

Freshly ground black pepper

⅔ cup freshly grated low-fat Parmesan cheese (or rice or soy cheese)

In a large saucepan, heat the oil over medium heat. Add the onion, celery, and carrots, and cook, stirring occasionally, until the vegetables soften, about 5 minutes.

Add the bay leaf, stock, and tomatoes, and bring to a boil. Reduce the heat to medium-low and simmer until the vegetables are tender, about 10 minutes.

Add the pasta and beans, and return the stock to a boil; then simmer over low heat, stirring constantly to prevent the pasta from sticking, until the pasta is cooked but not mushy, 8 to 15 minutes.

Add the spinach and cook for 2 minutes. Season with black pepper, sprinkle with cheese, and serve.

Per serving: 381.9 calories, 17.9 grams protein, 47 grams carbohydrates, 15.3 grams fat, 10.8 grams fiber

VEGETARIAN MAIN DISHES

These light and healthy stuffed peppers are great for all diet-free vegetarians. Serve them with ½ to ⅔ cup of beans (such as black, navy, or kidney) to make a complete fat-burning meal.

1 tablespoon extra-virgin olive oil

1 large red onion, sliced

1 zucchini, diced

4 ounces mushrooms, sliced

1 clove garlic, crushed

1 (14-ounce) can chopped tomatoes with their liquid

1 tablespoon tomato paste

4 large yellow bell peppers

Scant ⅓ cup pine nuts

2 tablespoons chopped fresh basil

Freshly ground black pepper

½ cup finely grated low-fat Cheddar cheese (or soy or rice cheese)

Fresh basil leaves, for garnish

Preheat the oven to 350°F.

Heat the oil in a large saucepan over low heat. Add the onion, zucchini, mushrooms, and garlic, and cook for 3 minutes.

Stir in the tomatoes and tomato paste, bring to a boil, and simmer over medium-low heat uncovered, stirring occasionally, until thickened slightly, 10 to 15 minutes.

Cut the bell peppers in half lengthwise and seed them. Blanch in a large pot of boiling water for 3 minutes, then drain and dry.

Remove the vegetable mixture from the heat, stir in the pine nuts and chopped basil, and season with black pepper. Set aside.

Place the bell peppers in a shallow ovenproof dish, cut side up, and fill with the vegetable mixture.

Cover the dish with foil and bake for 20 minutes. Uncover, sprinkle with the cheese, season with more black pepper, if using, and bake uncovered for

5 to 10 minutes more, until the cheese is melted and bubbling. Garnish with fresh basil leaves and serve.

Per serving: 254.5 calories, 12.6 grams protein, 24.7 grams carbohydrates, 14 grams fat, 5.8 grams fiber

Fresh, raw veggies on a whole wheat Sandwich Thin and topped with hummus makes a perfect vegetarian sandwich. A side of black beans makes it a fat-burning meal guaranteed to help you maximize fat loss.

½ cup black beans, rinsed and drained

1 whole wheat Sandwich Thin

2 tablespoons prepared hummus

1 cup fresh spinach leaves, stemmed

2 slices soy cheese

2 slices green or red bell pepper

1 slice tomato

Warm the beans in a small saucepan over medium-low heat.

Spread 1 tablespoon of hummus on each half of the Sandwich Thin. Cover one half with all the remaining ingredients, except the beans, and top with the other half. Serve with the beans on the side.

Per serving: 321 calories, 20.1 grams protein, 47.8 grams carbohydrates, 7.7 grams fat, 12.7 grams fiber

VEGETARIAN MAIN DISHES

Spicy Spinach Pizza

This rich and savory pizza is topped with a colorful and tasty arrangement of hot peppers, sun-dried tomatoes, fresh spinach, onions, and cheese.

2 tablespoons extra-virgin olive oil

1 or 2 fresh hot peppers, seeded and finely chopped

1 onion, chopped

2 cloves garlic, chopped

10 sun-dried tomatoes in oil, drained and roughly chopped

1 (14-ounce) can tomatoes with their liquid, chopped

1 tablespoon tomato paste

Freshly ground black pepper

8 cups spinach leaves, stemmed and chopped

1 large (8- to 9-inch) whole wheat pita

1 cup soy cheese, grated

Heat 1½ tablespoons of the oil over medium heat in a large saucepan. Add the hot peppers, onion, and garlic, and cook until the onion is soft and golden, about 5 minutes. Be careful not to burn the garlic or it will taste bitter.

Add the sun-dried tomatoes, canned tomatoes, and tomato paste. Season with black pepper and simmer over medium-low heat, uncovered, stirring occasionally, for 15 minutes.

Stir the spinach into the sauce and cook, stirring, until the spinach has wilted and there is no excess moisture, 5 to 10 minutes. Remove from the heat and set aside to cool.

Preheat oven to 425°F.

Brush the pita with the remaining ½ tablespoon of the oil, and spoon the sauce over it. Sprinkle evenly with the cheese, and bake for 12 to 15 minutes, or until crisp and golden. Serve immediately.

Per serving: 410 calories, 21.3 grams protein, 44.3 grams carbohydrates, 19.9 grams fat, 9.7 grams fiber

VEGETARIAN MAIN DISHES

This squash recipe makes a fat loss plate solo. Or cut your portion in half and have it as a snack.

1 tablespoon extra-virgin olive oil

2 (2½ pounds total) summer squash

2 large onions

6 tablespoons light butter

1 can Campbell's Healthy Request cream of chicken soup

1 cup shredded low-fat cheese (or rice or soy cheese)

1 cup light sour cream

1 (2-ounce) jar pimientos, drained

1 package Pepperidge Farm stuffing mix

Preheat the oven to 350°F. Spray a 9 × 13 inch ovenproof casserole with nonstick cooking spray.

In a large skillet, heat the oil over medium heat and sauté the squash and onions, 4 to 6 minutes. Drain and transfer to the prepared casserole. Stir in the butter, soup, cheese, sour cream, pimientos, and half the stuffing mix. Top with the remaining stuffing mix and bake until brown, about 30 minutes.

Per serving: 388.8 calories, 15 grams protein, 44.6 grams carbohydrates, 17.8 grams fat, 6 grams fiber

VEGETARIAN MAIN DISHES

Stuffed Veggie Quesadillas

Serve this Mexican favorite with your choice of salsa and a side of beans for a gooey and delicious fat-burning meal.

½ cup chopped red and green bell peppers

¼ tomato, chopped

2 tablespoons chopped onion (optional)

½ cup chopped mushrooms

5 cups spinach leaves, stemmed and chopped

½ cup sliced zucchini

2 large low-carb whole wheat tortillas

½ cup canned artichoke hearts, rinsed and drained

½ cup shredded cheese blend (or rice or soy cheese)

1 cup cooked black beans (or other beans of your choice)

4 tablespoons prepared salsa

Spray a large skillet with nonstick cooking spray, and sauté the bell peppers, tomato, onion (if using), mushrooms, spinach, and zucchini over medium heat until soft, 3 to 5 minutes. Set aside and keep warm.

Spray another skillet with nonstick cooking spray. Place 1 tortilla in the pan, and layer with the sautéed vegetables, artichoke hearts, and cheese. Cover with the second tortilla.

Cook over medium heat until the bottom is golden, about 2 minutes, then flip the quesadilla and cook until the cheese is melted.

Warm the beans in a small saucepan over medium-low heat. Cut the quesadilla in half, and serve each half with 2 tablespoons of salsa and ½ cup of beans.

Per serving: 393 calories, 33.6 grams protein, 56 grams carbohydrates, 12 grams fat, 28.3 grams fiber

VEGETARIAN MAIN DISHES

A Tangy Vegetarian Sandwich

MAKES 1
SERVING

Piled high with fresh vegetables, topped with cheese, spread with tangy honey mustard, and served with ½ cup of beans to boost your protein, this sandwich makes an outstanding fat-burning meal.

1 teaspoon honey mustard

1 whole wheat Sandwich Thin or whole wheat pita

¼ cup spinach leaves, stemmed and chopped

2 slices of medium tomato

¼ cup chopped cucumber

½ tablespoon shredded carrot

1 slice low-fat provolone cheese (or rice or soy cheese)

¼ cup alfalfa sprouts

Spread the honey mustard on both halves of the Sandwich Thin. Arrange the spinach, tomato, cucumber, carrot, cheese, and alfalfa sprouts on the bottom half, and top with the other half.

Per serving: 259 calories, 13.4 grams protein, 29.2 grams carbohydrates, 12.1 grams fat, 12.8 grams fiber

VEGETARIAN MAIN DISHES

Veggie-Nut Terrine

This is equally delicious straight from the oven or out of the fridge. Serve it with a side salad to complete your fat-burning meal.

1 pound broccoli, cut into florets

1 tablespoon extra-virgin olive oil

1¼ cups sliced raw almonds

1 cup fresh whole wheat bread crumbs

¼ cup plain nonfat Greek yogurt

4 tablespoons low-fat Parmesan cheese (or rice or soy cheese)

Freshly ground black pepper

Pinch of freshly grated nutmeg

2 egg whites, lightly beaten

8 cups spinach leaves, stemmed

8 tablespoons balsamic vinaigrette

Preheat the oven to 350°F. Lightly grease a 9 × 5 × 3 inch loaf pan.

Pan-fry the broccoli over medium heat until tender, 3 to 4 minutes. Drain and reserve ¼ of the smallest florets. Chop the rest finely.

In a large bowl, combine the almonds, bread crumbs, yogurt, and Parmesan cheese. Season with black pepper and nutmeg. Gradually stir in the chopped broccoli, reserved florets, and egg whites. Spoon the mixture into the prepared pan.

Place the loaf pan in a roasting pan, and fill the outer pan with boiling water till it comes halfway up the sides of the loaf pan. Bake the terrine for 20 to 25 minutes. Remove the loaf pan from the oven, being mindful of any dripping hot water. Dry off the loaf pan, turn the terrine out onto a serving plate, and cut it into 4 equal slices.

Toss the spinach with the vinaigrette, and divide the salad into 4 equal servings.

Per serving: 343.8 calories, 20.2 grams protein, 32.7 grams carbohydrates, 16.8 grams fat, 11 grams fiber

VEGETARIAN MAIN DISHES

**MAKES 1
SERVING**

This dressing not only tastes great but also slows the conversion of carbs into blood sugar, which helps maximize fat loss.

¼ cup apple cider vinegar

2 tablespoons freshly squeezed lemon juice

1 tablespoon extra-virgin olive oil

½ tablespoon salt-free Mrs. Dash original blend

½ teaspoon freshly ground black pepper

Combine all ingredients and mix well.

Per serving: 136 calories, 0.3 grams protein, 5.3 grams carbohydrates, 14 grams fat, 0.5 grams fiber

VEGETARIAN MAIN DISHES

Spicy Black Beans

(V)

A slow-carb side to keep you burning fat.

1 tablespoon extra-virgin olive oil

1 medium onion, sliced

2 medium green bell peppers, cored, seeded, and cut into ½-inch-wide strips

4 large cloves garlic, chopped

1 teaspoon ground cumin

2 (15-ounce) cans black beans, drained

⅓ cup water

½ teaspoon hot red pepper flakes

3 tablespoons chopped fresh cilantro

Freshly ground black pepper

Heat the oil in a medium sauté pan over medium heat. Add the onion and bell peppers and sauté for 5 minutes. Turn the heat to low, and add the garlic and cumin. Cook, stirring, for 1 minute.

Add the beans, water, and red pepper flakes. Raise the heat to medium-high, stir, and bring to a boil. Cover and simmer over medium-low heat for 5 to 8 minutes, or until the bell peppers are tender.

Stir in the cilantro, and season with black pepper.

Per serving: 246 calories, 13.6 grams protein, 40.6 grams carbohydrates, 4.2 grams fat, 16 grams fiber

Serve either version of these beans with Mamma Approved Corn Bread (page 239) for just the right amount of protein and carbs to keep you burning fat.

**WHOLE BEANS
MAKES 2
SERVINGS**

**REFRIED BEANS
MAKES 1
SERVING**

For whole beans

2 cups dried beans (pinto, black, Peruvian)

Salt

For refried beans

2 tablespoons extra-virgin olive oil, or more, as desired

1 cup cooked beans (pinto, black, Peruvian)

Bean cooking water as needed

Minced garlic (optional)

Make whole beans: Wash and pick through the beans to remove dirt and stones. Place the beans in a large saucepan, cover with water, and bring to a boil over medium-high heat. Boil until beans are soft, then season with salt.

Make refried beans: Heat the oil in a large frying pan over medium heat, and add the beans. Stir and toss for 3 to 4 minutes, adding bean water to flavor and moisten the beans to your taste. With a potato masher, mash the beans until they resemble mashed potatoes, adding more bean water as needed.

For additional flavor, add the garlic to taste. For a creamier texture and flavor, add a bit more oil.

Per serving for whole beans: 227 calories, 15.2 grams protein, 40.8 grams carbohydrates, 15 grams fat, 0.9 grams fiber

Per serving for refried beans: 467 calories, 15.2 grams protein, 40.8 grams carbohydrates, 28.9 grams fat, 15 grams fiber

SIDE DISHES

MAKES 8 SERVINGS

The ginger and soy sauce in this slow-carb recipe brings Chinese restaurant taste right into your kitchen.

8 cups broccoli florets

1 teaspoon finely grated fresh gingerroot

2 tablespoons low-sodium soy sauce

2 tablespoons rice vinegar

1 teaspoon evaporated cane juice (see note on page 145)

1½ tablespoons water

1½ tablespoons extra-virgin olive oil

Freshly ground black pepper

Bring a large pot of water to a boil over medium-high heat. Add the broccoli and cook until crisp-tender, 3 to 5 minutes. Drain well, and transfer to a shallow serving dish.

Meanwhile, in a small bowl, combine the ginger, soy sauce, vinegar, cane juice, water, and oil, and season with black pepper. Whisk until well blended, and drizzle it over the broccoli.

Per serving: 54.5 calories, 1 gram protein, 4.5 grams carbohydrates, 2.5 grams fat, 2 grams fiber

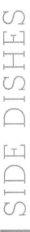

SIDE DISHES

Grilling cauliflower gives it a whole new taste sensation. Coated with spiced melted butter to enhance the tenderness brought out by the grill, this slow-carb dish is great with any meal.

MAKES 4 SERVINGS

¾ cup low-sodium chicken broth

1 tablespoon light butter

1 tablespoon chopped garlic

½ teaspoon dry mustard

¼ teaspoon crushed red pepper flakes

1 head cauliflower

Preheat the grill to medium-high.

In a small skillet, combine the broth, butter, garlic, mustard, and red pepper flakes, and cook over high heat, stirring, until reduced to ¼ cup, 5 to 10 minutes.

Trim the leaves from the cauliflower, and cut the core from the underside of the head, making sure not to cut so deep that the head falls apart. Tear off a piece of heavy-duty foil large enough to enclose the entire head of cauliflower. Place it shiny side up on a work surface, and put the cauliflower in the middle, turning up the sides of the foil to almost enclose it. Pour the reduced broth mixture over the cauliflower, and seal the foil packet. Set it on the grill grate, cover the grill, and cook 25 to 40 minutes, rotating the packet but not turning it over, until the cauliflower is just tender when pressed with a gloved finger.

To serve, open the foil and cut the cauliflower into bite-size pieces.

Per serving: 55.8 calories, 4 grams protein, 8.6 grams carbohydrates, 1.5 grams fat, 3.7 grams fiber

SIDE DISHES

MAKES 4 SERVINGS

Serve this slow carb with a protein and a fast carb to make a complete fat-burning meal.

1 tablespoon Dijon mustard

½ cup plain nonfat Greek yogurt

1 tablespoon freshly squeezed lemon juice

½ teaspoon balsamic vinegar

2 teaspoons extra-virgin olive oil

2 teaspoons water

4 cups shredded savoy cabbage or 4 cups packaged coleslaw mix

Freshly ground black pepper

In a small bowl, combine the mustard, yogurt, lemon juice, vinegar, oil, and water until blended. Place the cabbage in a large serving bowl and toss with the dressing. Season with black pepper.

Per serving: 52.8 calories, 3.8 grams protein, 5 grams carbohydrates, 4.6 grams fat, 2.8 grams fiber

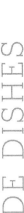

SIDE DISHES

This tangy slow-carb combo is sure to spice up any meal.

**MAKES 4
SERVINGS**

1 medium red bell pepper, cored and seeded

2 medium green bell peppers, cored and seeded

4 green onions, green parts only

1 tablespoon extra-virgin olive oil

½ teaspoon chili paste

½ teaspoon minced garlic

2 teaspoons low-sodium soy sauce

2 tablespoons low-sodium vegetable broth

Cut the bell peppers into 1-inch-wide strips and then in half crosswise. Cut the wide ends of the scallion tops in half lengthwise, and then cut into 1-inch lengths.

Heat the oil in a heavy skillet or wok over high heat. Add the bell peppers, and sauté 2 minutes. Reduce the heat to medium, cover, and cook 4 minutes more, stirring often.

Add the scallions, chili paste, garlic, soy sauce, and broth. Cover and cook until the peppers are tender, 1 to 2 minutes.

Per serving: 65 calories, 1.1 grams protein, 5.5 grams carbohydrates, 4 grams fat, 1.6 grams fiber

SIDE DISHES

MAKES 8 SERVINGS

Plantains, a staple of the Cuban diet, look a lot like bananas but taste very different. This recipe can be used to cook up a fast carb for a fat-burning meal or a delicious snack.

8 medium green plantains

4 tablespoons plantain cooking water

2 tablespoons extra-virgin olive oil

2 tablespoons minced garlic

Cut the ends off the unpeeled plantains and discard. Put the rest of the plantains in a large pot of boiling water over medium-high heat, and boil until the skin slips off. Transfer the plantains to a large bowl, discarding the skins, and mash them, adding 4 tablespoons of the hot cooking water to help soften the fruit. Add the oil and garlic, and continue to mash the plantains until they reach your desired consistency.

Per serving: 160.8 calories, 0.8 grams protein, 31.2 grams carbohydrates, 27.2 grams fat, 2.3 grams fiber

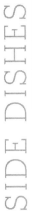

SIDE DISHES

Here's a great grilled zucchini recipe to serve as a slow carb.

1½ pounds medium zucchini or yellow summer squash

2 tablespoons Italian-style vinaigrette dressing

Salt and freshly ground black pepper

3 tablespoons freshly grated Parmesan cheese (or rice or soy cheese)

Preheat a grill pan over medium-high heat.

Trim the ends of the zucchini, and then cut them lengthwise into 4 spears each. Place the spears in a baking dish, and coat them on all sides with the dressing. Sprinkle with salt and black pepper to taste.

Transfer the zucchini to the grill pan, skin side down, and cook about 10 minutes, turning to brown them on all sides, until crisp-tender. Sprinkle with the cheese, cover, and cook until the zucchini is tender and the cheese has formed a crust, 2 to 3 minutes.

Per serving: 76.3 calories, 3.5 grams protein, 11.2 grams carbohydrates, 2.7 grams fat, 3.4 grams fiber

SIDE DISHES

MAKES 3 SERVINGS

Each little pancake is filled with protein-rich ingredients that create a delicious snack or the slow-carb portion of a meal. Enjoy them with a small salad and your favorite dressing.

3½ cups coarsely grated peeled zucchini

⅔ cup freshly grated Parmesan cheese (or rice or soy cheese)

4 egg whites, beaten

4 tablespoons whole wheat flour

Freshly ground black pepper

Squeeze the zucchini in a clean dish towel to remove any excess liquid.

In a bowl, combine the zucchini with the cheese, egg whites, and flour, and season with black pepper.

Spray a large frying pan with nonstick cooking spray and heat over medium heat. Using 2 tablespoons of the zucchini mixture for each pancake, cook 3 at a time until golden, 2 or 3 minutes on each side. Remove from the pan and keep warm while cooking the rest. You should end up with 12 pancakes.

Per serving: 177 calories, 15.2 grams protein, 16.6 grams carbohydrates, 6.2 grams fat, 4.2 grams fiber

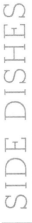

SIDE DISHES

This vegetarian chili is great when served with ¼ cup brown rice and ¼ cup plain nonfat Greek yogurt to complete a fat-burning meal.

MAKES 4 SERVINGS

2 onions, chopped

1 clove garlic, crushed

3 celery stalks, chopped

1 green bell pepper, diced

1 cup sliced mushrooms

1 (14-ounce) can kidney beans, rinsed and drained

1 (14-ounce) can chopped tomatoes with their liquid

⅔ cup tomato sauce

2 tablespoons tomato paste

1 tablespoon ketchup

1 teaspoon hot chili powder

1 teaspoon ground cumin

1 teaspoon ground coriander

Freshly ground black pepper

Combine the onions, garlic, celery, bell pepper, and mushrooms in a large saucepan, and mix well.

Stir in the kidney beans, tomatoes, tomato sauce, tomato paste, and ketchup.

Add the chili powder, cumin, and coriander; season with black pepper; and mix well.

Place the pan over medium-high heat, cover, and bring to a boil. Lower the heat and simmer, stirring occasionally, until the vegetables are tender, 20 to 30 minutes.

Per serving: 171.5 calories, 10.1 grams protein, 33.9 grams carbohydrates, 1.4 grams fat, 9.3 grams fiber

SIDE DISHES

MAKES 5 SERVINGS

Serve this cold soup with your preferred protein for a complete fat-burning meal.

2 red bell peppers, quartered lengthwise

1 yellow bell pepper, quartered lengthwise

2 small zucchinis, trimmed and quartered lengthwise

1 red onion, cut into ½-inch-thick slices

1 teaspoon extra-virgin olive oil

3 large tomatoes, cored and chopped

1 clove garlic, peeled

½ teaspoon dried oregano

1 cup water

¼ cup shredded basil leaves

1 tablespoon red wine vinegar

Salt and freshly ground black pepper

Preheat the grill to medium.

Grill the bell peppers, skin-side toward the flame, until the skin is blackened, 5 to 10 minutes. Place in a paper bag and set aside for 15 minutes.

Meanwhile, brush the zucchini and onion slices with the oil, and grill or broil until well browned and tender, about 5 minutes. Chop the browned vegetables coarsely and set aside.

Remove the peppers from the bag and rub off the charred skin. Coarsely chop the yellow pepper, then set it aside with the reserved zucchini and onions.

Place the red peppers in a food processor or blender with the tomatoes, garlic, and oregano, and puree until smooth. Transfer to a bowl and stir in the water, basil, vinegar, and reserved chopped vegetables.

Add a dash each of salt and black pepper. Cover and refrigerate until cool, about 30 minutes.

Per serving: 71.2 calories, 2.92 grams protein, 14.08 grams carbohydrates, 1.58 grams fat, 3.92 grams fiber

SIDE DISHES

**MAKES 4
SERVINGS**

Two summertime favorites, basil and berries, combine to make a fabulous fat-burning meal when served with your favorite protein.

3 tablespoons extra-virgin olive oil

3 tablespoons balsamic vinegar

⅛ teaspoon freshly ground black pepper

8 cups torn romaine lettuce

3 cups sliced strawberries

½ cup chopped Texas sweet onion (optional)

¼ cup chopped fresh basil

Combine the oil, vinegar, and pepper in a large bowl, and whisk to combine.

Add the lettuce, strawberries, onion (if using), and basil. Toss gently and serve immediately.

Per serving: 179.8 calories, 2.9 grams protein, 18.6 grams carbohydrates, 10.1 grams fat, 6.5 grams fiber

SIDE DISHES

Potatoes with a Zing

Tired of the same old baked potatoes? With the addition of some herbs and spices, you can transform your favorite fast carb into something even tastier.

2 large baking potatoes

1 teaspoon sunflower oil

1 small onion, finely chopped

1 (1-inch) piece fresh gingerroot, grated

1 teaspoon ground cumin

1 teaspoon ground cilantro

½ teaspoon ground turmeric

4 tablespoons plain nonfat Greek yogurt

Preheat the oven to 375°F.

Prick the potatoes with a fork and bake for 1 hour, or until soft. Cut the potatoes in half, and carefully scoop out the flesh, keeping the skins intact. Set the flesh and skins aside.

Heat the oil in a nonstick frying pan over medium heat, and sauté the onion for a few minutes until softened. Stir in the ginger, cumin, cilantro, and turmeric. Stir over low heat for about 2 minutes, then add the potato flesh.

Cook the potato mixture for another 2 minutes, stirring occasionally. Spoon the mixture into the potato skins, and top each potato half with a tablespoon of yogurt.

Per serving: 106.3 calories, 3.2 grams protein, 21 grams carbohydrates, 1.3 grams fat, 3.2 grams fiber

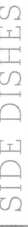

Serve this tangy potato salad with your favorite protein to make a festive fat-burning meal.

For the salad

2 pounds small red potatoes

¾ pound yellow squash, cut lengthwise into ½-inch slices

⅛ teaspoon freshly ground black pepper

For the dressing

⅓ cup chopped fresh chives

3 tablespoons chopped fresh flat-leaf parsley

2 tablespoons chopped fresh basil

1 tablespoon chopped fresh tarragon

¼ teaspoon grated lemon zest

3 tablespoons freshly squeezed lemon juice

2 tablespoons water

2 tablespoons extra-virgin olive oil

2 tablespoons finely chopped cornichons

⅛ teaspoon freshly ground black pepper

Make the salad: Place the potatoes in a large saucepan, cover with water, and bring to a boil over medium-high heat. Reduce the heat and simmer for 18 minutes, or until the potatoes are tender. Drain, cut the potatoes into quarters, and place them in a large bowl.

Preheat the grill to medium heat.

Lightly coat the squash with nonstick cooking spray, and season with the black pepper. Grill until brown and tender, 2 minutes on each side. Add to the potatoes.

Make the dressing: Mix all the ingredients in a small bowl, and whisk to combine. Pour the dressing over the potato mixture and toss gently. Serve the salad warm or chilled.

Per serving: 170.5 calories, 4 grams protein, 41.2 grams carbohydrates, 7.3 grams fat, 5.5 grams fiber

SIDE DISHES

Red Sweet Potatoes

Enjoy these tender, tasty sweet potatoes with your favorite protein and slow carb.

4 medium red-skinned sweet potatoes

2 tablespoons extra-virgin olive oil

½ teaspoon granulated garlic

¼ cup low-fat sour cream

¼ teaspoon hot paprika

Preheat the grill to medium-high.

Slice the potatoes, skin on, into ½-inch rounds, and place them in a resealable plastic bag. Drizzle in the oil and sprinkle with the garlic. Seal the bag, leaving some air inside, and toss gently to coat the potatoes.

Grill the potato slices, turning frequently, until fork-tender and showing grill marks, 10 to 12 minutes. Remove the potatoes from the grill and arrange on a large, warm platter. Spoon a small amount of sour cream on top of each potato and sprinkle with the paprika.

Per serving: 155.2 calories, 3 grams protein, 23.8 grams carbohydrates, 5.6 grams fat, 2.2 grams fiber

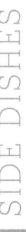

SIDE DISHES

These yams are definitely full of sugar and spice and everything nice!

MAKES 10 SERVINGS

4 pounds yams or sweet potatoes

4 egg whites

4 tablespoons brown sugar

4 tablespoons light butter, melted

1 teaspoon ground cinnamon

⅛ teaspoon ground allspice

⅛ teaspoon ground nutmeg

½ cup chopped pecan halves

Pierce the potatoes with a fork in several places. Cook in the microwave on high for about 20 minutes, or until cooked through. Cool, remove the skins, and put the flesh in a large bowl.

Preheat the oven to 375°F.

Mash the potatoes until smooth, and then beat in the egg whites one at a time, blending thoroughly after each addition. Stir in 2 tablespoons of the brown sugar; 2 tablespoons of the melted butter; and the cinnamon, allspice, and nutmeg. Beat until the mixture is light and fluffy.

Transfer the potato mixture to an ungreased 3-quart casserole dish. Arrange the pecans in a single layer on top. Sprinkle with the remaining brown sugar and drizzle with the remaining melted butter.

Bake for 25 minutes, or until browned and bubbly.

Per serving: 151.1 calories, 2.9 grams protein, 17.6 grams carbohydrates, 8.2 grams fat, 2.8 grams fiber

SIDE DISHES

Basmati Coconut Rice

Some people seem to think that when you're trying to reduce your waistline, you shouldn't be eating "white" foods. That's a silly notion—and unfortunate for those who give up dishes as delicious as this one.

1 cup white basmati rice

1 cup light coconut milk (organic if possible)

2 teaspoons brown sugar

2½ cups water

½ cup sweetened flaked coconut, lightly toasted

Combine the rice, coconut milk, and brown sugar in a bowl. In a medium saucepan over high heat, bring the water to a boil, add the rice mixture, and cover and simmer over low heat until done, 15 to 20 minutes. Stir in the coconut flakes just before serving.

Per serving: 135.3 calories, 2.3 grams protein, 24 grams carbohydrates, 3.3 grams fat, 0 grams fiber

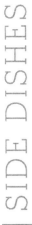

SIDE DISHES

This signature dish is a delicious accompaniment to a lean steak, grilled chicken, or any Mexican entrée. Browning the rice with onions and garlic before cooking it in chicken stock makes this fast-carb favorite even more delectable.

2 tablespoons extra-virgin olive oil

2 cups medium- or long-grain brown rice

1 onion, finely chopped

1 clove garlic, minced

3 cups low-sodium chicken or vegetable broth

1 cup diced fresh or canned tomatoes, strained

Pinch of dried oregano

In a large skillet over medium-high heat, heat the oil; add the rice, and cook until it browns, a few minutes. Add the onion and garlic, and cook, stirring frequently, until the onion is soft, about 4 minutes.

In a saucepan, bring the broth to a simmer over low heat. Add the tomatoes and oregano, add the rice mixture, and bring to a simmer. Cover, lower the heat, and cook 15 to 25 minutes, depending on the type of rice and the instructions on the package. Turn off the heat and let the rice sit covered for 5 minutes.

Per serving: 133 calories, 7 grams protein, 17.5 grams carbohydrates, 5.3 grams fat, 1.7 grams fiber

SIDE DISHES

Fat Loss Mac 'n' Cheese

When the ingredients are blood sugar friendly and the nutrients are balanced, you can have a fast carb like mac 'n' cheese and your fat loss, too.

2½ cups uncooked elbow macaroni

1¾ cups soymilk

4 tablespoons light butter, melted

2 tablespoons all-purpose unbleached white flour

½ teaspoon freshly ground black pepper

2 whole eggs and 2 egg whites, beaten

2½ cups low-fat shredded Cheddar cheese (or rice or soy cheese)

1 slice whole wheat bread, ground into bread crumbs

Cook the macaroni according to package directions, drain, and set aside.

Preheat the oven to 350°F.

Combine the soymilk and 3 tablespoons of the melted butter in a mixing bowl; add the flour, black pepper, and eggs and egg whites; and whisk until smooth.

Spray a shallow 2-quart baking dish with nonstick cooking spray. Layer half the cooked macaroni in the bottom of the dish; sprinkle with 2 cups of the cheese, and top with the remaining macaroni. Pour the milk and egg mixture over the macaroni. Toss the bread crumbs with the remaining 1 tablespoon of butter and sprinkle over the top. Bake the macaroni and cheese uncovered for 45 to 50 minutes. Sprinkle with the remaining ½ cup of cheese and bake about 5 minutes longer.

Per serving: 290 calories, 16 grams protein, 24 grams carbohydrates, 14.5 grams fat, 2.3 grams fiber

SIDE DISHES

This delicious Italian sauce comes with 15 grams of protein. Serve it with your choice of pasta (1 cup cooked for women; 1¼ cups for men).

MAKES 8 SERVINGS; ½ CUP PER SERVING

- 2 tablespoons light butter
- 2 tablespoons unbleached all-purpose white flour
- 4 cups soymilk or skim milk, warmed
- 1 cup freshly grated Parmesan cheese (or rice or soy cheese)
- 1 teaspoon garlic powder

Make a roux by combining the butter and flour in a saucepan over medium heat and cooking it, stirring, until the mixture is thickened but not browned or burned, about 2 minutes. Add half the milk and whisk until smooth. Add the remaining milk and heat slowly.

Add the cheese and garlic powder, and cook slowly, stirring with a spatula from the bottom so that it doesn't burn, until the cheese is incorporated and the sauce is smooth. Strain if necessary to remove any burned particles.

Per serving: 200 calories, 15 grams protein, 9 grams carbohydrates, 11 grams fat, 0 grams fiber

SIDE DISHES

This fat-burning twist on traditional stuffing is designed to enhance any Thanksgiving feast. And you don't have to wait for Thanksgiving to enjoy it.

1 (1-pound) loaf sliced whole wheat bread

¾ cup light butter

1 onion, chopped

4 celery stalks, chopped

2 teaspoons poultry seasoning

Freshly ground black pepper

1 cup low-sodium chicken broth

Let the bread air-dry for 1 to 2 hours, then trim off the crusts and cut into cubes.

In a Dutch oven, melt the butter over medium heat. Cook the onion and celery in the butter until soft. Add the poultry seasoning and black pepper to taste, then stir in the bread cubes until evenly coated. Add the chicken broth and mix well.

Chill for 1 to 2 hours, then reheat in a 350°F oven for 10 to 15 minutes before serving.

Per serving: 181.4 calories, 5.5 grams protein, 24.1 grams carbohydrates, 7.3 grams fat, 4 grams fiber

BREAKFASTS, SNACKS, AND DESSERTS

Crispy Peach Parfait

MAKES 2 SERVINGS

When in a hurry, this delicate dish is easy to whip up. The combination of Greek yogurt, peaches, and oats topped with a fruity jam makes a delicious breakfast.

- 1 peach or nectarine, pitted and cut in small cubes
- 1 cup Kashi Heart to Heart honey-toasted oat cereal
- 2 (5.3-ounce) containers plain nonfat Greek yogurt or ⅔ cup plain low-fat yogurt
- 1 tablespoon no-sugar-added fruit jam of your choice
- 1 tablespoon unsweetened fruit juice of your choice

Divide the fruit equally between two tall glasses, reserving a few cubes for decoration. Sprinkle ½ cup cereal over the fruit in each glass, and top each with half of the yogurt.

In a separate bowl, stir together the jam and juice. Top the parfaits with the mixture, garnish with the reserved fruit, and serve.

Per serving: 222 calories, 17.1 grams protein, 39.7 grams carbohydrates, 1.5 grams fat, 5.1 grams fiber

Fiery Tofu Scramble

This vegetarian mixture of spicy peppers, diced onions, jalapeños, and tofu makes a tasty and satisfying fat-burning snack.

1 tablespoon extra-virgin olive oil

1 cup diced onion

1 medium jalapeño, seeded and diced*

½ green bell pepper, diced

1 red bell pepper, diced

1 teaspoon low-sodium soy sauce

½ teaspoon turmeric

1 cup prepared salsa (optional)

1 (12.3-ounce) package firm silken tofu

In a large skillet, heat the oil over medium-low heat, add the onion, and cook, stirring often, until softened, about 3 minutes. Stir in the hot and bell peppers, soy sauce, turmeric, and salsa, if using. Cook for 2 minutes, and then crumble the tofu into the skillet. Stir and cook until warmed through, 5 minutes more.

Per serving: 184 calories, 12.2 grams protein, 15.6 grams carbohydrates, 8.4 grams fat, 3.1 grams fiber

---

*For a spicier dish, keep the seeds.

BREAKFASTS, SNACKS, AND DESSERTS

This frittata makes a great breakfast, but you could also enjoy it for either lunch or dinner.

2 cups chopped broccoli

¾ cup chopped tomato

¼ cup corn kernels (organic if possible)

½ cup low-fat shredded Cheddar cheese (or rice or soy cheese)

1 (16-ounce) carton egg whites

2 whole eggs

1 tablespoon water

Salt-free Mrs. Dash original blend

Preheat the oven to 400°F. Spray a 9 × 9 inch square baking pan with nonstick cooking spray.

Layer the broccoli, tomatoes, corn, and cheese over the bottom of the pan. Beat the egg whites and whole eggs with the water, and pour the egg mixture over the broccoli mixture in the pan. Sprinkle with the seasoning mix to taste, and bake uncovered for 30 minutes, or until the eggs are completely set.

Per serving: 314 calories, 38.2 grams protein, 20.5 grams carbohydrates, 9.25 grams fat, 4.2 grams fiber

BREAKFASTS, SNACKS, AND DESSERTS

Chocolate and bananas are a classic combination, and these muffins are laced with an extra boost of protein powder to keep you burning fat.

6 tablespoons light soymilk

3 egg whites

10 tablespoons light butter, melted

1 cup whole wheat flour

1 cup protein powder

1 teaspoon baking powder

¾ cup evaporated cane juice (see note on page 145)

4 ounces semisweet chocolate chips

2 small bananas, mashed

Preheat the oven to 400°F. Line 12 large muffin cups with paper muffin cups.

Combine the soymilk, egg whites, and butter in a bowl, and whisk well.

In a separate bowl, mix together the flour, protein powder, and baking powder. Add the cane juice and chocolate chips, and stir to combine. Slowly stir in the milk mixture, but do not beat it. Fold in the mashed bananas.

Spoon the batter into the muffin cups and bake for 20 minutes, or until golden. Allow to cool before removing the muffins from the tin.

Per serving: 166.6 calories, 10 grams protein, 29.2 grams carbohydrates, 7.6 grams fat, 2.3 grams fiber

This traditional American favorite can be combined with your favorite slow carb and protein to make a fat-burning meal or eaten as a snack on its own.

MAKES 8 SIDE-DISH OR 16 SNACK SERVINGS

½ cup unbleached all-purpose flour

½ cup whole wheat flour

1 cup yellow cornmeal*

⅔ cup evaporated cane juice (see note on page 145)

1 teaspoon salt

3 teaspoons baking powder

1 whole egg

1¼ cups soymilk or nonfat milk

⅓ cup light butter

Preheat the oven to 400°F. Spray a 9-inch round cake pan with nonstick cooking spray.

In a large bowl, combine the flours, cornmeal, cane juice, salt, and baking powder. Stir in the egg, soymilk, and butter just until combined.

Pour the batter into the prepared pan and bake for 22 to 26 minutes, or until a toothpick inserted into the center comes out clean.

Per serving, for 8 servings: 300 calories, 5.6 grams protein, 44.5 grams carbohydrates, 12.3 grams fat, 2.2 grams fiber

Per serving, for 16 servings: 150 calories, 2.8 grams protein, 22.3 grams carbohydrates, 6.1 grams fat, 1.1 grams fiber

BREAKFASTS, SNACKS, AND DESSERTS

---

*Arrowhead Mills brand is recommended.

Shrimp with Apple Salsa

**MAKES 4
SERVINGS**

This is just the right amount of cooked shrimp, juicy apples, peppers, and onions to complete a fat-burning snack for four.

For the salsa

½ cup diced apple

¼ cup diced red onion

¼ cup diced red bell pepper

2 tablespoons minced fresh cilantro

2 tablespoons apple juice

2 tablespoons red wine vinegar

Pinch of chipotle pepper powder

For the shrimp

6 tablespoons hot paprika

2 tablespoons freshly ground black pepper

1 tablespoon chili powder

2 teaspoons brown sugar

Pinch of cayenne

32 medium shrimp, peeled, deveined, and butterflied

1 tablespoon extra-virgin olive oil

Make the salsa: Combine the salsa ingredients in a medium bowl; mix well, and refrigerate for at least 1 hour.

Make the shrimp: Preheat the grill to medium-high.

Combine the paprika, black pepper, chili powder, brown sugar, and cayenne in a small bowl. Lightly dust the shrimp with the spice mix. Brush the grill rack with the oil, and grill the shrimp until pink, about 1 minute per side.

Serve the shrimp with the salsa.

Per serving: 148 calories, 12 grams protein, 15 grams carbohydrates, 6.2 grams fat, 6 grams fiber

Ⓥ

With the right ingredients and method, you can enjoy fried green tomatoes and still keep your body in fat-burning mode. This snack is one of my childhood favorites! Serve the tomatoes with my Delicious Dipping Sauce (page 243).

¼ cup all-purpose unbleached white flour

¼ cup whole wheat flour

⅛ teaspoon cayenne

Salt and freshly ground black pepper

4 large green tomatoes, cut into ¼-inch-thick slices for a total of 32 slices

1 cup low-fat buttermilk

½ cup cornmeal

¼ cup extra-virgin olive oil

In a medium bowl, combine the flours, cayenne, salt, and black pepper. Dust the tomato slices on both sides with the flour mixture, then dip them in the buttermilk and dust them with the cornmeal.

Heat the oil in a medium nonstick skillet over medium-high heat. Add the tomatoes and cook, turning, until light golden brown on both sides. Remove the tomatoes from the pan and drain on paper towels. Serve the tomatoes as is or with the dipping sauce.

Per serving: 130 calories, 5 grams protein, 16.7 grams carbohydrates, 8 grams fat, 2.1 grams fiber

BREAKFASTS, SNACKS, AND DESSERTS

Power Chowder

This chowder makes a perfect fat-burning snack.

3 ears corn, shucked

3 red bell peppers, halved

4 large tomatoes, halved and seeded

1 tablespoon extra-virgin olive oil

4 cups chopped onion (about 2 medium)

3 (14-ounce) cans fat-free, low-sodium chicken or vegetable broth

¼ teaspoon freshly ground black pepper

¼ cup crumbled low-fat blue cheese (or rice or soy cheese)

2 tablespoons chopped fresh chives

Preheat the grill to medium-high.

Place the corn and the bell peppers, skin side down, on a grill rack. Grill 5 minutes, turning the corn occasionally. Add the tomatoes, cut side down, and grill just until slightly charred, 30 to 60 seconds. Remove the vegetables from the heat and let them cool for 10 minutes.

Coarsely chop the tomatoes and bell peppers, and place them in a medium bowl. Cut the corn kernels off the cobs and add them to the tomato mixture.

In a large saucepan, heat the oil over medium heat. Add the onions and sauté, stirring occasionally, until tender, about 7 minutes. Add the broth and the grilled vegetables, increase heat to high, and bring to a boil. Reduce the heat and simmer until the vegetables are tender, about 30 minutes. Remove from the heat and cool for 20 minutes.

Transfer a third of the soup to a blender and process until smooth; transfer to a large bowl and repeat the process twice with the remaining soup. Wipe the saucepan with a paper towel and press the pureed mixture through a sieve back into the pan. Discard the solids. Place the pan over medium heat until the chowder is heated through. Taste and season with the black pepper.

Measure about 1½ cups of chowder into each of 6 bowls, and top each serving with 2 teaspoons of cheese and 1 teaspoon of chives.

Per serving: 136 calories, 14.5 grams protein, 19.6 grams carbohydrates, 5.7 grams fat, 4.2 grams fiber

BREAKFASTS, SNACKS, AND DESSERTS

1 cup light mayonnaise

1 tablespoon freshly squeezed lemon juice

1 tablespoon minced capers

1 tablespoon minced onion

1 teaspoon Dijon mustard

1 teaspoon horseradish

1 teaspoon hot paprika

4 sprigs fresh cilantro or flat-leaf parsley, chopped

½ teaspoon Worcestershire sauce

Blend all the ingredients and refrigerate until ready to serve.

Per serving: 70 calories, 0 grams protein, 1 gram carbohydrates, 7 grams fat, 0 grams fiber

MAKES 8 SERVINGS

BREAKFASTS, SNACKS, AND DESSERTS

MAKES 8 SERVINGS

Imagine enjoying a slice of angel food cake topped with vanilla custard for a snack and still reducing your waistline! Well, no need to imagine anymore; just try this fat loss dessert.

1½ cups soymilk

¼ cup evaporated cane juice (see note on page 145)

4 large eggs

1 tablespoon vanilla extract

8 (2-ounce) slices angel food cake

Place the soymilk in a microwave-safe bowl and microwave on high for 3 minutes.

Whisk the cane juice and eggs together in a medium microwave-safe bowl. Gradually add the hot soymilk, whisking continuously. Microwave the mixture on high for 2½ minutes, stirring once halfway through.

Stir in the vanilla, cover, and cool to room temperature.

Divide the custard equally over the cake slices and serve.

Per serving: 167 calories, 8.5 grams protein, 34 grams carbohydrates, 3.2 grams fat, 1.5 grams fiber

BREAKFASTS, SNACKS, AND DESSERTS

Have one of these cinnamony treats whenever your sweet tooth is calling for satisfaction.

For the dough

1 (¼-ounce) package active dry yeast

½ cup warm water

½ cup scalded skim or soymilk

¼ cup evaporated cane juice (see note on page 145)

⅓ cup light butter, melted

2 egg whites

3½ to 4 cups whole wheat flour

For the filling

½ cup melted light butter

¾ cup evaporated cane juice

2 tablespoons ground cinnamon

For the glaze

4 tablespoons light butter

2 cups powdered sugar

1 teaspoon vanilla extract

3 to 6 tablespoons hot water

Make the dough: In a small bowl, dissolve the yeast in the warm water and set aside until the yeast bubbles. In a large bowl, combine the milk, cane juice, butter, and egg whites. Add 2 cups of the flour and mix until smooth. Add the yeast mixture, and mix in more of the flour until the dough is easy to handle. Knead the dough on a lightly floured surface for 5 to 10 minutes. Place it in a well-greased bowl, cover, and let it rise until doubled in bulk, 1 to 1½ hours.

When doubled in size, punch down the dough, then roll it out on a floured surface into a 17 × 9 inch rectangle.

Spray the bottom of a 17 × 14 inch baking pan with nonstick cooking spray.

Make the filling: Spread the butter over the dough. Combine the cane juice and cinnamon, and sprinkle it over the top. Beginning at one long side, roll up the dough, and pinch the edges to seal the roll. Cut the roll into 17 (1-inch-thick) slices.

Preheat the oven to 350°F.

Place the cinnamon rolls close together in the pan and set aside to rise until the rolls have doubled in size, about 45 minutes.

Bake the cinnamon rolls for about 30 minutes, or until nicely browned. Set aside to cool slightly while you make the glaze.

Make the glaze: Mix together the butter, sugar, and vanilla. Add the water, 1 tablespoon at a time, until the glaze reaches a spreadable consistency. Spread it over the slightly cooled rolls.

Per serving: 194.6 calories, 7.9 grams protein, 33.9 grams carbohydrates, 5.6 grams fat, 3.1 grams fiber

These are great just as they are, but you can add a bit more ginger to the recipe if you wish to make the gingery taste pop even more.

½ cup brown sugar

6 tablespoons light butter, softened

¼ cup sugar-free syrup, sweetened with Splenda, if available

¼ cup molasses

7 tablespoons light soymilk

2 egg whites, beaten

1½ cups chickpea flour

2 teaspoons ground ginger

1 teaspoon ground cinnamon

1½ teaspoon baking powder

Preheat the oven to 325ºF. Line a 13 × 4 × 4 inch loaf pan with parchment paper, and spray it with nonstick cooking spray.

Combine the sugar, butter, syrup, and molasses in a saucepan over medium heat, stirring occasionally until melted and blended. Remove from the heat and cool slightly, then mix in the soymilk and egg whites.

In a large bowl, combine the flour, ginger, cinnamon, and baking powder. Slowly mix the wet ingredients into the flour mixture.

Pour the batter into the prepared pan and bake for 1½ hours, or until firm to the touch and lightly browned.

Cool in the pan for a few minutes, and then turn out onto a wire rack to cool completely. Cut into 10 equal rectangles and store in an airtight container or wrapped in foil.

Per serving: 150.4 calories, 4.1 grams protein, 25.3 grams carbohydrates, 4.3 grams fat, 1.5 grams fiber

BREAKFASTS, SNACKS, AND DESSERTS

MAKES 8 SERVINGS

Satisfy your sweet tooth with juicy berries, rich Greek yogurt, and delightful shortcakes. You can freeze any extras and have them on hand for the next time you crave sweets.

4 cups blueberries

1 cup plus 4 tablespoons Splenda

1 tablespoon freshly squeezed lime juice

1 cup whole wheat pastry flour

1 cup all-purpose unbleached flour

1 tablespoon baking powder

6 tablespoons light butter

3 tablespoons minced crystallized ginger

¾ cup soymilk or nonfat milk

1 egg white

1 tablespoon water

⅓ cup plain nonfat Greek yogurt

1 teaspoons arrowroot powder or cornstarch

Preheat the oven to 400°F.

Combine the blueberries, 3 tablespoons of the Splenda, and the lime juice in a medium saucepan over medium-low heat. Cook, stirring frequently, until the berries begin to pop, about 3 minutes. Remove from the heat and set aside.

Combine the flours and baking powder in a food processor, and pulse three times. Add the butter and ginger, and pulse until the mixture resembles coarse meal. Place the flour mixture in a large bowl and add the soymilk, stirring until moist. Transfer the dough to a lightly floured surface and form it into a 7-inch circle. Then cut it into 8 wedges. Place the wedges 1 inch apart on a baking sheet. Combine the egg white and water in a small bowl, and lightly brush the wedges with the mixture. Sprinkle evenly with 1 tablespoon of the Splenda.

Bake for 20 minutes, or until the shortcakes are golden brown. Cool on a wire rack.

BREAKFASTS, SNACKS, AND DESSERTS

Place the Greek yogurt in a medium bowl, and beat at medium speed until soft peaks form.

Place the remaining 1 cup of Splenda and the arrowroot in a blender or food processor and blend on high speed for 1 minute, until the texture resembles powdered sugar. Scrape down the bowl as needed. Add the Splenda mixture to the yogurt, beating until stiff peaks form. Split the shortcakes in half horizontally; spoon ⅓ cup berry mixture over each bottom, top each with 1½ tablespoons of the yogurt, and cover each with a shortcake top.

Per serving: 268.4 calories, 6.6 grams protein, 45 grams carbohydrates, 7.9 grams fat, 4.9 grams fiber

**MAKES 8
SERVINGS**

This cake is not only delicious but also gluten-free. Moist to the taste and easy on the waist is how I describe this nutritious and delicious recipe!

2 large oranges

2 cups ground raw almonds

1 egg white

3 whole eggs

¾ cup sugar-free brown rice syrup or maple syrup

1 teaspoon baking soda

¼ teaspoon salt

Preheat the oven to 275°F. Lightly grease a 9-inch round cake pan.

Wash the whole oranges and place them in a large pot with enough water to cover them. Boil over high heat for 90 minutes, or until soft.

Place the whole oranges in a food processor and blend until smooth. Add all the remaining ingredients and blend until smooth.

Pour the batter into the prepared pan and bake for 45 to 50 minutes, or until a toothpick inserted in the center comes out clean.

Per serving: 193.6 calories, 8.2 grams protein, 12.8 grams carbohydrates, 13.9 grams fat, 3.6 grams fiber

BREAKFASTS, SNACKS, AND DESSERTS

Crunchy Cookies with a Chocolate Swirl

These vanilla cookies coated in chocolate and almonds will show your friends how fabulous a fat-burning dessert can be.

MAKES 32 COOKIES, 1 COOKIE PER SERVING

1½ cups all-purpose unbleached flour

1½ cups whole wheat flour

1 cup evaporated cane juice (see note on page 145)

½ teaspoon baking powder

1 cup light butter, cut into small cubes and chilled

½ cup light soymilk

2 teaspoons vanilla extract

12 ounces semisweet chocolate chips

1 teaspoon solid vegetable shortening

1 cup sliced raw almonds

Heat the oven to 375°F. Line a baking pan with foil, leaving several inches of foil overhanging on the shorter sides. Lightly coat the foil with nonstick cooking spray.

In a large bowl, whisk together the flours, cane juice, and baking powder. Add the butter and work it into the flour mixture with a fork until the mixture resembles cornmeal.

Drizzle the soymilk and vanilla over the butter-flour mixture and toss lightly. The dough will be dry and crumbly. Firmly press the crumbly dough into the prepared baking pan in an even layer.

Bake for 25 to 28 minutes, or until firm and golden brown around the edges. Let the cookie slab cool in the pan until set. Then, using the foil, lift the cookie from the baking pan and transfer it to a wire rack to cool completely.

Cut the slab into 16 squares, then cut each square into 2 triangles and place them on wax or parchment paper.

In a microwave-safe bowl, combine the chocolate and shortening. Microwave on high for 15-second intervals, stirring between each, until melted and smooth.

BREAKFASTS, SNACKS, AND DESSERTS

One at a time, dip each edge of each cookie in the melted chocolate to create a frame of chocolate around the cookie. Then dip each edge of each cookie in the almonds, pressing gently so that the nuts stick to the chocolate. Transfer the finished cookies to a sheet of wax paper to harden. The cookies can be stored in an airtight container at room temperature up to 4 days.

Per serving: 153.8 calories, 2.4 grams protein, 22.4 grams carbohydrates, 7.1 grams fat, 1.2 grams fiber

Two of these outrageous cookies make for a perfectly sweet fat-burning snack!

MAKES 18 SERVINGS, 2 COOKIES PER SERVING

⅓ cup light butter, at room temperature

½ cup evaporated cane juice (see note on page 145)

2 egg whites

½ teaspoon vanilla extract

1 cup whole wheat flour

1 teaspoon baking powder

⅛ teaspoon baking soda

½ cup semisweet chocolate chips

18 marshmallows

6 ounces dark chocolate

Preheat the oven to 350°F. Spray a large baking sheet with nonstick cooking spray.

In a small mixing bowl, cream the butter and evaporated cane juice together until light and fluffy. Beat in the egg whites and vanilla.

In another bowl, combine the flour, baking powder, and baking soda. Gradually beat the flour mixture into the egg-white mixture. Stir in the chocolate chips.

Scoop out tablespoon-size portions of dough to form 36 balls. Place them on the prepared baking sheet about 2 inches apart. Bake for 8 minutes.

While the cookies bake, cut each marshmallow in half crosswise with kitchen shears.

Remove the cookies from the oven, but leave the oven on. Quickly place 1 marshmallow half, cut-side down, on top of each hot cookie. Return the cookies to the oven and bake 1 to 2 minutes longer, or just until the marshmallows begin to puff. Remove the cookies from the oven, cool 2 minutes, transfer the cookies to a wire rack, and gently flatten each marshmallow with your fingers.

Melt the dark chocolate in the top of a double boiler over hot but not boiling

BREAKFASTS, SNACKS, AND DESSERTS

water. Spoon about 1 teaspoon of melted chocolate over each marshmallow. Let the s'mores stand until the chocolate sets, about 30 minutes.

Per serving: 141.5 calories, 2.4 grams protein, 22.9 grams carbohydrates, 6 grams fat, 3.3 grams fiber

Before you toss out that cold coffee left in the pot, think about making this warm mocha treat.

- ½ cup unsweetened cocoa powder
- 2 tablespoon arrowroot powder or corn starch
- 2 cups soymilk, or skim or low-fat milk
- 2 tablespoons brown rice syrup or honey (organic if possible)
- 2 tablespoons brewed coffee or 1 teaspoon instant coffee dissolved in 2 tablespoons hot water
- 1 teaspoon vanilla extract

In a saucepan, whisk together the cocoa and arrowroot, then stir in the soymilk and syrup. Bring to a boil over medium heat, stirring constantly until the mixture boils and thickens, 6 to 8 minutes.

Remove the saucepan from the heat, and stir in the coffee and vanilla. Whisk until cooled.

Pour into two individual custard cups and chill for several hours before serving.

Per serving: 174 calories, 10.8 grams protein, 35.2 grams carbohydrates, 5 grams fat, 8.2 grams fiber

MAKES 4 SERVINGS

If you want something more than a piece of apple pie, give this scrumptious treat a try.

BREAKFASTS, SNACKS, AND DESSERTS

4 large baking apples

1 small banana, chopped

¼ cup orange-flavored sweetened dried cranberries, chopped*

2 tablespoons honey (organic if possible)

¾ teaspoon ground cinnamon

4 tablespoons freshly squeezed orange juice

Generously core each apple to allow adequate space for the chopped fruit. Peel a strip off the top of each apple. Place each apple in a 6-ounce ramekin or custard cup.

Combine the banana, cranberries, honey, and cinnamon in a medium bowl. Fill the apples evenly with the fruit mixture, and pour 1 tablespoon of orange juice over each apple.

Cook in the microwave on medium heat until soft, 5 to 7 minutes. Let stand 5 minutes before serving.

Per serving: 198.3 calories, 0.9 grams protein, 52.3 grams carbohydrates, 0.6 grams fat, 6.6 grams fiber

_____

*Use regular dried cranberries if you can't find the orange-flavored fruit.

No one would ever guess that this combination of apples and blackberries covered in freshly squeezed orange juice and topped off with cinnamon and sugar makes a fat-burning snack or dessert.

MAKES 8 SERVINGS

For the fruit

1 pound cooking apples

1 cup blackberries

Juice and grated zest of 1 orange

⅓ cup light brown sugar

For the topping

1½ cups whole wheat flour

1 tablespoon light butter, cut in small pieces

⅓ cup evaporated cane juice (see note on page 145)

1½ tablespoons ground cinnamon

Preheat oven to 400°F. Spray a 5-cup baking dish with nonstick cooking spray.

Make the fruit: Peel and core the apples, then slice them into the prepared baking dish. Level the surface, and scatter the blackberries on top. Sprinkle the orange zest and brown sugar evenly over the top of the fruit, then pour the juice over all. Set the fruit mixture aside.

Make the topping: Sift the flour into a bowl, add the butter, and combine with a fork until the mixture resembles coarse bread crumbs. Stir in the cane juice and cinnamon. Scatter the topping over the fruit, pressing it around the edges of the dish to seal in the juices.

Bake for 30 to 35 minutes, or until the crumble is golden.

Per serving: 181.8 calories, 3.6 grams protein, 42.5 grams carbohydrates, 1.2 grams fat, 4.5 grams fiber

BREAKFASTS, SNACKS, AND DESSERTS

Note to Readers

If you're pleased with the results you've achieved so far and would like to learn more about how to stay lean and diet-free for life, please visit my website (www.dietfreelife.com) to learn more about my seminars and workshops, the Diet-Free for Life Challenge, the Detox Drop Kits and program, daily diet-free support by text and email, and other online fat loss tools.

Index

Page numbers in **bold** indicate tables; those in *italics* indicate photographs; and those followed by "n" indicate notes.